100 Grey Cases Paediatrics

for MRCPCH

Nagi Giumma Barakat MB BCh, MRCPCH, MSc Epilepsy, CCST
Consultant Paediatrician
Hillingdon Hospital
and Honorary Consultant Paediatric Neurologist
Great Ormond Street Hospital
UK

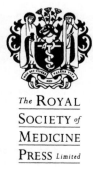

The ROYAL
SOCIETY *of*
MEDICINE
PRESS *Limited*

© 2003 Royal Society of Medicine Press Ltd

Published by the Royal Society of Medicine Press Ltd
1 Wimpole Street, London W1G 0AE, UK
Tel: +44 (0)20 7290 2921
Fax: +44 (0)20 7290 2929
E-mail: publishing@rsm.ac.uk
Website: www.rsmpress.co.uk

British Library Cataloguing in Publication Data
A catalogue record for this book is available from the British Library

ISBN 1-85315-524-1

Distribution in Europe and Rest of World:
Marston Book Services Ltd
PO Box 269
Abingdon
Oxon OX14 4YN, UK
Tel: +44 (0)1235 465500
Fax: +44 (0)1235 465555

Distribution in the USA and Canada:
Royal Society of Medicine Press Ltd
c/o Jamco Distribution Inc
1401 Lakeway Drive
Lewisville, TX 75057, USA
Tel: +1 800 538 1287
Fax: +1 972 353 1303
E-mail: jamco@majors.com

Distribution in Australia and New Zealand:
MacLennan + Petty Pty Ltd
Suite 405, 152 Bunnerong Road
Eastgardens NSW 2036
Australia
Tel: + 61 2 9349 5811
Fax: + 61 2 9349 5911

Phototypeset by Phoenix Photosetting, Chatham, Kent
Printed and bound in Great Britain by Bell and Bain Ltd, Glasgow

Contents

Preface

This book is designed to help candidates preparing for the MRCPCH Part II in the UK and Ireland. Great effort has been made to make the cases in the book as close as possible to the latest exam questions. It has features which are not found in many other books, e.g. all cases are real cases of mine, collected over the last 10 years, while I was in training or working as a paediatrician in the UK. The cases are varied and I have tried to avoid repetition. This book was written and designed to be helpful to paediatricians in training or working in hospitals. Many cases have added features such as neuroimaging, X-rays, EEGs etc.

The cases included in this book cover all the subspecialties in paediatrics but most are on paediatric neurology. The discussion of cases is kept simple, comprehensive and clinically oriented. Much of the explanation reflects my personal experiences and opinions. Many sources are used in the discussion sections, including textbooks, journals, the Internet, and courses. Most of the figures are from my personal collection.

This book is intended for use not only for the MRCPCH written exam, but also for the viva, short and long cases. Using this book will also give guidance to candidates on how to answer questions. This book will facilitate and enhance candidate knowledge in paediatric medicine. It is practical and easy to use, and I hope you will enjoy using it.

NGB

Dedication

To all my colleagues and teachers who attended or taught me at the faculty of Medicine, Garryounis University-Benghazi-Libya between 1977 and 1984. To my teachers in the UK who helped to train me in paediatrics and paediatric neurology. To my wife Lobna and daughters Iman, Nadia, and Yasmine who inspired my thoughts to write this book.

Acknowledgements

Special thanks are given to all colleagues who helped me to obtain some of the photographs presented in this book and allowed me to use them. I also thank my wife, who helped me to edit this book as well as looking after our daughters. Special thanks to the RSM team, Peter Richardson and Nora Naughton, who have helped me and been very patient, even though I did not manage to deliver the final manuscript on time.

Abbreviations

AA	Amino acids
ABG	Arterial blood gas
ACTH	Adrenocorticotrophic hormone
AD	Autosomal dominant
ADEM	Acute disseminated encephalomyelitis
AED	Anti-epileptic drugs
Alb	Albumin
Alk. Ph	Alkaline phosphatase
ALL	Acute lymphoblastic leukaemia
ALT	Alanine transaminase (alanine aminotransferase)
ANA	Anti-nuclear antibodies
AO	Aorta
AR	Autosomal recessive
AS	Aortic stenosis
ASD	Atrial septal defect
ASOT	Anti-streptolysin-O-titres
AST	Aspartate transaminase (aspartate aminotransferase)
AV	Arterio-venous malformation
AXR	Abdominal X-ray
BC	Blood culture
BCG	Bacillus Calmette – Gaérin
Be	Base excess
BILLI	Bilirubin
BM	Basal metabolic rate
BMI	Body mass index
BPD	Broncho-pulmonary dysplasia
BRECH	Benign Rolandic epilepsy of childhood
BS	Blood sugar
C3	Complement
Ca	Calcium
CF	Cystic fibrosis
CFM	Cerebral function monitoring
CH50	Complement 50
CK	Creatinine kinase
Cl	Chloride
CLD	Chronic lung disease
CMPI	Cow's milk protein intolerance
CMV	Cytomegalovirus
CO_2	Carbon dioxide
CPAP	Continuous positive airway pressure
Cr	Creatinine
CRP	C-reactive protein
C/S	Culture/sensitivity
CSA	Child sexual abuse
CSF	Cerebrospinal fluid
CSS	Continuous spike and sharp wave
CT	Computerised tomography
CXR	Chest X-ray
DCT	Direct Coombs test
DDVAP	Desamino-dearginine-vasopressin
DIC	Disseminated intravascular coagulation

DMSA	Dimercaptosuccinic acid
DNA	Diribonucleic acid
DW	Diffuse weight imaging
E	Eosinophils
EBV	Epstein–Barr virus
ECG	Electrocardiograph
ECHO	Echocardiograph
EEG	Electroencephalograph
ELSCS	Elective caesarean section A
EMG	Electromyography
ERG	Electroretinograph
ESR	Erythrocyte sedimentation rate
ETT	Endotracheal tube
EVP	Evoked visual potential
FBC	Full blood count
Fib	Fibrinogen
FME	Forensic medical examiner
FSH	Follicle-stimulating hormone
FTND	Full term normal delivery
FTT	Failure to thrive
γGT	Gamma-glutamyltransferase
GAG	Glycosated aminoglycans
GFR	Glomerular filtration rate
GH	Growth hormone
GIT	Gastrointestinal tract
Glu	Glucose
GN	Glomerulonephritis
GOR	Gastro-oesophageal reflux
Hb	Haemoglobin
HBC	Hepatitis C serology
HbF	Haemoglobin F
HBsA	Hepatitis B surface antibodies
HBSag,	Hepatitis B surface antigen
HbF	Fetal haemoglobin
HbSS	Sickle-cell disease
HCO_3	Bicarbonate
Hct	Haematocrit
HIE	Hypoxic ischaemic encephalopathy
HMD	Hyaline membrane disease
HR	Heart rate
HSV	Herpes simplex virus
HUS	Haemolytic uraemic syndrome
HVA	Homovanillic acid
Ig	Immunoglobulin
IM	Intramuscularly
INR	International normalised ratio
IPPV	Intermittent positive partial ventilation
IUGR	Intrauterine growth retardation
IVC	Inferior vena cava
IVH	Interventricular haemorrhage
IVIG	Intravenous immunoglobulin
IVP	Intravenous pyelograph
K	Potassium
KUB	Kidney, ureters, bladder
L	Lymphocytes
LA	Left atrium

LBBB	Left bundle branch block
LFT	Liver function test
LH	Luteinising hormone
LP	Lumbar puncture
LV	Left ventricle
M	Monocytes
MAG3	
MAP	Mean arterial pressure
MCA	Middle cerebral artery
MCAD	Methylmalonic Co-A deficiency
MCAI	Middle cerebral artery infarct
MCHC	Mean corpuscular haemoglobin concentration
MCV	Mean corpuscle volume
Mg,	Magnesium
MIBG	*Meta*-iodobenzylguanidine
mmHg	Millimetres of mercury
MRA	Magnetic resonance arteriography
MRI	Magnetic resonance imaging
MS	Multiple sclerosis
MSU	Midstream urine
N	Neutrophils
Na	Sodium
NA1	Non-accidental injuries
NBT	Nitro blue test
NCPAP	Nasal continuous positive airway pressure
NCS	Nerve conduction study
NEC	Necrotising enterocolitis
NGT	Nasogastric tube
NH_4	Ammonia
NPA	Nasopharyngeal aspirate
O_2	Oxygen
OFC	Occipto-frontal circumference
OT	Occupational therapy
PA	Pulmonary artery
Pb	Lead
PCP	*Pneumocystis carinii* pneumonia
PCR	Polymerase chain reaction
PCV	Packed cell volume
PDA	Patent ductus arteriosus
PEEP	Peak end-expiratory pressure
PEFR	Peak expiratory flow rate
PET	Positron emission topography
PHH	Post-haemorrhagic hydrocephalus
PICU	Paediatric intensive care unit
PLT	Platelets
Pro	Protein
PT	Prothrombin time
PTT	Partial thromboplastin time
RA	Right atrium
RBBB	Right bundle branch block
RBC	Red blood cells
Ret	Reticulocytes
RNA	Ribonucleic acid
RR	Respiratory rate
RV	Right ventricle
s	Second

Sat	Saturation
SCBU	Special care baby unit
SCID	Severe combined immune deficiency
SIDS	Sudden infant death syndrome
SLE	Systemic lupus erythematosus
SSPE_	Subacute sclerosing panencephalitis
SVC	Superior vena cava
SVT	Supraventricular tachycardia
SXR	Skull X-ray
T_4	Thyroid hormone
TAPVD	Total anomaly pulmonary venous drainage
TB	Tuberculosis
TFT	Thyroid function test
TGA	Transposition of great arteries
TIBC	Total iron body capacity
TIBC	Total iron body capacity
TS	Tuberous sclerosis
TSH	Thyroid-stimulating hormone
TT	Thrombin time
TV	Tidal volume
U	Urea
UAC	Umbilical catheter artery
Ur	Urea
U&E	Urea and electrolytes
URTI	Upper respiratory tract infection
US	Ultrasound
UTI	Urinary tract infection
UVC	Umbilical venous catheter
VC	Vital capacity
VEP	Visually evoked potential
VIIIc	Factor eight C
VLCF-	Very long chain fatty acids
VMA	Vanillylmandelic acid
VSD	Ventricular septal defect
VUR	Vesicoureteral reflux
WAS	Wiskott–Aldrich syndrome
WCC	White cell count

Case 1

A 13-year-old girl presented to Accident and Emergency (A&E) with a history of lethargy, joint pain and cough. Both of her parents are from Jamaica. Her problem started 1 month ago, with an upper respiratory tract infection (URTI). She was seen by her family doctor, and a viral infection was diagnosed. She had a past history of rashes on her body, but her family doctor never saw them. On examination, she has palpable cervical lymph nodes of various sizes, a congested throat, generalised myalgia and a swollen ankle joint on the left side. Her BP is 120/75 mmHg, HR 90 b.p.m. and RR 22/min. A urine test showed protein + with red cells. Other test results are:

Hb	9.7 g/dl
WCC	$4 \times 10^9/l$ with neutropenia and lymphopenia
PLT	$100 \times 10^9/l$
Ret	2.6%
CRP	20

1. Which three other important investigations should be carried out?
2. What treatments should you prescribe?
3. What are three possible differential diagnoses?

She was admitted for further investigation and on the second night, her oxygen requirement increased to 3 l/min via a facemask to maintain a Sat level above 93%. All cultures were negative.

4. Which single investigation should you carry out?

Her condition got worse, she was transferred to the paediatric intensive care unit (PICU), she required ventilation, and other procedures were carried out. Her blood pressure remained high (130/90 mmHg) and she was treated with nifedipine. A kidney US scan was reported as normal, as was a hormonal study. She was treated with antibiotics for 7 days. A viral titre shows IgG for EBV. A Mantoux test is very weakly positive, although she had never received a BCG.

5. Which three other investigations may help the diagnosis?
6. What other treatment should be added at this stage?

Case 2

An infant baby girl aged 36 months was seen in A&E with a history of vomiting and diarrhoea for the previous 3 days. In the last 24 hours, she became irritable and grew pale. She is not interested in eating but is still drinking fluids. She was born full term and has no previous problems. The family lives in a council flat without central heating. The father is a heavy smoker and the mother is heavily pregnant. The infant looks pale with a peripheral capillary refill rate of 3 s. Her HR is

140 b.p.m., RR 30/min and BP 90/60 mmHg. Her liver is 3 cm below the right costal margin, the right kidney is palpable and there is no jaundice. Her urine shows protein +, RBC ++ and no organisms or leukocytes. All cultures are negative.

1. List four immediate investigations
    a   ESR
    b   INR
    c   Renal US with Doppler
    d   Urea and electrolytes (U&E)
    e   Hepatitis B and C serology
    f   Full blood count (FBC)
    g   24-hour urinary protein
    h   VMA
    i   Renal biopsy
2. What is the most likely diagnosis?
    a   Haemolytic uraemic syndrome (HUS)
    b   UTI
    c   Gastroenteritis
    d   Obstructive renal failure
    e   Right renal artery thrombosis
    f   Right renal vein thrombosis
    g   Wilms' tumour
    h   Acute glomerulonephritis
3. Name three steps of management.

Case 3

An 11-year-old boy was referred to A&E with a history of limping and pain in his right leg. The day before, he was chasing his sister, fell and hit the side of the coffee table, and has since been complaining of pain in his right knee. There is no family history of any illnesses apart from his aunt, who died 3 years ago with an illness described as a stroke, after a long time of unspecified illness.

Systemic and general examinations were reported as normal, except for a slight proximal weakness of the right leg.

1. What one test should you carry out?
    a   ESR
    b   CRP
    c   Right and left knee X-ray
    d   Right knee X-ray
    e   Right knee US
    f   Right knee MRI
    g   Right knee CT

The boy presented 5 days later with more weakness and was seen by the orthopaedic surgeon, who diagnosed muscle weakness and referred him to the paediatrician, who would see him in 2 days. The same night he came back to A&E with more weakness in his right leg and a right arm that felt 'heavy'. There is marked weakness of the proximal muscle groups in the right upper and lower limbs. The reflexes are present and the sensation is intact.

2. Which three differential diagnoses are correct?
    a   Guillain–Barré syndrome
    b   Myeloencephalitis
    c   Myositis
    d   Spinal cord injury
    e   Sciatic nerve injury
    f   Hemiplegia secondary to intercerebral insult
    g   Dysraphism
    h   MS
    i   ADEM
3. What two abnormalities appear on his cranial MRI?

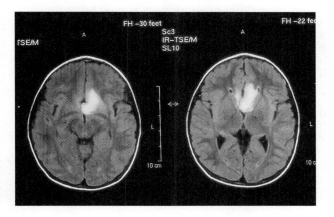

4. Which two investigations should be carried out?
    a   Nerve conduction study
    b   LP
    c   EMG
    d   Cranial MRI
    e   Muscle biopsy
    f   CK
    g   Lower limb muscle MRI
    After 2 days in hospital the boy started having difficulty in swallowing and was not able to use his right leg.
5. What is the diagnosis?

Case 4

Since the age of 3 years, this 7-year-old girl has presented with a history of recurrent mouth ulcers. She was born by a full-term normal delivery (FTND) and her mother said she is a healthy girl. Her mother has ulcers in her mouth from time to time but, not as many as her daughter. The girl eats a packed lunch every day, with only brown bread and a high-fibre diet. She has two siblings, who are healthy. Her bowel habit is normal. During the summer holidays her ulcers are less frequent and she may get them once only over a period of 8 weeks. She is currently a healthy young girl with one ulcer on the inner right side of her lower lip. The test results are:

Hb	10.2 g/dl
WCC	$7 \times 10^9/l$
PLT	$380 \times 10^9/l$
MCV	80 fl
MCHC	32 g/dl
LFT	Normal
Stool	Normal

1. Which three other investigations should be carried out and in what order
   a   ESR
   b   Upper GIT endoscopy with biopsy
   c   Endomyseal antibodies
   d   Stool for reducing substances
   e   Barium swallow
   f   Dental check
   g   Throat swab for *Candida*
   h   Ig and IgG subclass
2. Which two abnormalities are visible in the figure below?

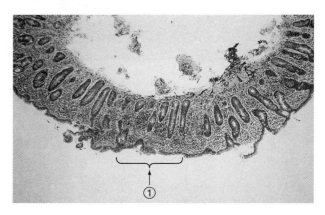

   a   Lymphocyte infiltration
   b   Total villous atrophy
   c   Partial villous atrophy
   d   Normal villi
   e   Granulomatous changes
   f   Crypts ulcers
3. What is the most likely diagnosis?

Case 5

A 6-week-old infant has a history of persistent cough and wheeze for 3 days. He is totally breastfed and feeding has become increasingly difficult in last 3 days. There is no history of whoop and he is afebrile. His birthweight was 3.5 kg and he now weighs 3.9 kg. His older sister had a febrile seizure at the age of 1 year. The family lives in a two-bedroomed flat and his father works as a builder. There has been no contact with anyone who has similar illness and there is no history of travel abroad.

The infant is active and has a Sat level of 92% in air.

He is using all his accessory muscles and there is no stridor.

Crackles were heard just before his cough and at the end of inspiration.

1.   Which two abnormalities appear on the CXR?

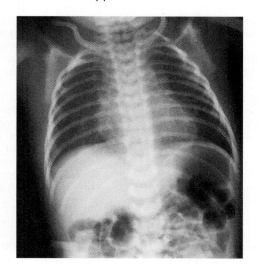

    a   Right upper lobe collapse
    b   Hyperinflation
    c   Increased bronchial airway thickening
    d   Left upper lobe collapse
    e   Large heart
    f   Fracture ribs 7 and 8
    g   Trachea deviated to right
    h   Right middle lobe cystic lesion

A throat swab shows *Haemophilus influenzae* and a pernasal swab is normal. Other test results are:

Blood gas	pH	7.29
	$PaCO_2$	5.2 kPa
	PaO_2	9 kPa
	HCO_3^3	17
	BE	−1

2. What is the abnormality on the arterial blood gas?
3. What one test can confirm the diagnosis?
    a   Sweat test
    b   NPA
    c   Pernasal swab
    d   Bronchoscopy and bronchial lavage
    e   Chest CT
    f   Ciliary motility study

Case 6

In a neonatal unit, there is a 13-day-old baby girl with floppiness, difficulty feeding and joint contractures. She was born following an easy pregnancy at 38 weeks' gestation by lower segment caesarean section due to a previous caesarean section. The baby cried immediately but half an hour later she became cyanosed and had difficulty in breathing. She was admitted to the special care baby unit (SCBU) and was ventilated for 8 days. Since then she has been fed by nasogastric tube (NGT) and has required oxygen via a facemask from time to time. Her mother has had two miscarriages. She has two older sisters, who are healthy, and there is no history of consanguinity or such an illness in the family. Another sister died at the age of 3 months, with a severe chest infection, and presented in a more severe state than she did. This sister required ventilation for 3 weeks, and was less alert, had joint contractures, clenched fists, hirsutism and was grossly floppy. Treatment was withdrawn and she died from chest infection.

On examination, this patient's occipital-frontal circumference (OFC) is on the 3rd centile, and she has short legs with contraction at the hips and knee joints. She has low-set ears, a large fontanelle, prominent skull suture and is less hairy than her sister. She is quite floppy, alert if she is awake, has no tongue fasciculation, and the gag reflex is present. There is some gravity movement in her limbs and reflexes are present but not brisk. The CK is 40 mmol/l (normal range: 42–60 mmol/l) and a metabolic screen is normal, which includes lumbar puncture (LP) and white cell enzymes, and there is no chromosomal abnormality.

An MRI scan of the brain was reported as normal and limb X-rays show no bony abnormality. Other systemic examinations are normal.

1. What is the most likely diagnosis?
    a   Congenital myotonic dystrophy
    b   Spinal muscle atrophy
    c   Congenital myasthenia gravis

    d   Arthrogryposis multiplexa
    e   Spina bifida
    f   Hereditary sensory motor neuropathy type 1
    g   Dysplasia punctatae congenital

2. List three further investigations in the order that they should be performed
    a   Tensilon test
    b   EMG
    c   NCS
    d   Muscle biopsy
    e   Cranial MRI
    f   Bone X-ray for bone density
    g   Skin biopsy

3. What management would you recommend?

Case 7

A 13-year-old boy presented to A&E with a history of abdominal pain, which was felt mainly on the right side of his abdomen. He is a keen footballer and played a game of football 2 days ago for about 2 hours. His pain was very sharp and radiated to his groin. No vomiting or diarrhoea occurred. The surgeon diagnosed appendicitis and asked for blood and urine tests to be carried out. He was admitted overnight and put on the next morning's operating list after review by a consultant surgeon. His urine test showed a RBC of more than 200 and no leukocytes. He slept overnight after being given ibuprofen but by 4.00 a.m. he started shouting as the pain got worse and was now spreading to his shoulders and back. Review was made by the surgeon, who prescribed more analgesia, and a request was made for the boy to remain nil-by-mouth in preparation for a possible appendectomy by the morning. After the ward round, an US of his kidneys and abdomen was organised, and it came back as normal. The paediatric team was asked to review the case, as he started complaining of spasms in his legs, arms, shoulder and said that they were painful. He was very irritable and jumpy when touched or talked to. He was started on antibiotics and acyclovir, and a brain CT scan was organised, which came back as normal, even with contrast. Other test results are:

Hb	13.3 g/dl
WCC	12×10^9/l (N 82%, L 3%)
PLT	150×10^9/l
LDH	1500 mmol/l
CK	6650 mmol/l
ALT	150 IU/l
Alk. Ph	990 IU/l
γGT	200 IU/l
Alb	37g/dl
Bilirubin	370 μmol/l (conjugated 15%)
ESR	30 mm/hour
CRP	12 after 2 weeks

The muscle spasms worsened and he was getting more agitated. Diazepam and chlormethiazole helped and he improved. All his viral serology was negative: *Mycoplasma* titres, Lyme disease, *Brucella* serology, and *Leptospirosis* IgM antibodies. He is fully vaccinated, with boosters at the age of 6 years and a BCG 1 year ago. He hasn't been abroad in the last 3 years and no one is ill at home. His urine still shows the presence of RBCs. His LP shows no abnormalities, even PCRs for bacteria and viruses. Tests for ANA and caeruloplasmine were negative. Screening for alpha-1-antitrypsin was negative. The lead level was also found to be normal.

1. Which other three tests may help the diagnosis?
    a   Brain MRI
    b   Muscle biopsy
    c   EMG
    d   NCS
    e   Repeat viral serology for EBV, parvovirus
    f   Repeat *Mycoplasma* titres
    g   DNA double strands
    h   Urine toxicology
2. What are three differential diagnoses?
    a   Viral hepatitis
    b   *Leptospirosis*
    c   Tetanus
    d   Meningoencephalitis
    e   Myositis
    f   Drug abuse
    g   Pancreatitis
    h   Systemic lupus erythematosus (SLE)

Case 8

An 18-month-old girl with a history of vomiting and poor weight gain was seen in A&E. She has not been very well in the last 3 months and in the last 6 months, after a URTI, she started to vomit and was not interested in feeding. She was born at 36 weeks' gestation by LSCS for polyhydramnios; there were no other concerns. She is hypotonic and her mother said that she has found it difficult to cope in the last 3 months with the frequency of changing her nappies and the large amount of fluid she is taking. Her general practitioner (GP) checked her blood sugar (BS), which was 4.5 mmol/l on three occasions. The renal scan shows nephrocalcinosis. There were no other illnesses and she is the first child in the family who has come from north Africa.

The child looks miserable; her weight is on the 10th centile, having dropped from the 50th. She is moderately dehydrated and her abdomen is soft, with no organomegaly. Her urine is clear and there is no metabolic problem, as all tests have been carried out in the past. Other test results are:

pH	7.56
PCO_2	4.2 kPa
PO_2	10 kPa
HCO_3	33
Be	1

1. What is the most likely diagnosis?
   a   Pyloric stenosis
   b   Protein cows' milk intolerance
   c   Lactose intolerance
   d   Bartter syndrome
   e   Cystic fibrosis (CF)
   f   Congenital adrenal hyperplasia
   g   Nephrogenic diabetes insipidus
2. Which two tests will help the diagnosis?

Case 9

A child presented with a history of recurrent wheeze and ear infections. He is now 2 years old and his wheezing episodes are under treatment with a regular budesonide inhaler and Bricanyl on a PRN basis. His ears are red and his left ear has a discharge. His mother said that this is the eighth ear infection he has had this year. Scattered wheeze was found on examination of his chest and there is no organomegaly. Other test results are:

Hb	13 g/dl
WCC	$20 \times 10^9/l$
N	70%
IgG	7 g/l (6.5–16 g/l)
IgE	19g/l (< 2 g/l)
Ear swab	*Pneumococcus*
Sweat Na	15 mmol/l (40–60 mmol/l)
CXR	Hyperinflated with bronchial thickening

1. What other one test should be carried out?
   a   Urine for protein
   b   Lymphocyte subsets
   c   Skin prick test
   d   IgG subclass
   e   NBT
   f   Stool for elastasis
   g   Hearing test
   h   DNA linkage study for Δ508
2. What are three appropriate steps in managing this child?
   a   Prophylactic antibiotics
   b   Bronchodilator
   c   Antihistamine nasal spray
   d   Grommet insertion
   e   Regular Ig transfusion
   f   Advice on allergy

g   Referral to dietitian
h   Regular inhaled corticosteroids for his asthma

Case 10

A 13-year-old child with a history of fever and lethargy subsequently developed mouth ulcers. There was no history of travel abroad. Her father is a heavy smoker, has recently had a productive cough and is under investigation. She said she feels hot all the time but has no cough or loss of weight. There is a tender, painful swelling on both lower limbs that appeared 2 days ago. Ibuprofen helped a lot, but the swelling, which looks like bruises, is still there. Her throat is mildly congested and a Mantoux test with 1:10 000 and 1:1000 is negative. The coeliac screen and ESR are also negative; the ESR is only 2. She started to menstruate 3 months ago, irregularly. She opens her bowel regularly and has had no previous health problem.

1. What are the three most likely diagnoses?
    a   Streptococcal throat infection
    b   Coxsackie virus A infection
    c   Coeliac disease
    d   SLE
    e   Crohn's disease
    f   Ulcerative colitis
    g   Tuberculosis
    h   Herpes gingival stomatitis
2. Which two investigations should be carried out and in what order?
    a   CXR
    b   Upper and lower GIT endoscopy
    c   Throat swab
    d   ANA
    e   Gastric aspirate for culture
    f   ASO titres
    g   *Mycoplasma* titres

ANSWERS 1–10

Case 1

1. a   Blood film
    b   ESR
    c   *Mycoplasma* titres
2. a   i.v. antibiotics
    b   Ibuprofen
3. a   Juvenile chronic arthritis (JCA)
    b   *Mycoplasma* infection
    c   Viral infection
4. CXR
5. a   DNA double strand

   b   Pleural fluid cytology
   c   Lymph node biopsy
6. a   Steroids
   b   NSAID

Systemic lupus erythematosus

SLE is a multisystem disease with many manifestations. Patients with SLE can be presented with many different symptoms and signs, and a high index of suspicion should be kept in mind for patients who present with multiorgan involvement.

The commonest presenting symptom is joint swelling and looks like JCA. Skin rashes vary from a butterfly rash on the face to purpura, urticaria or just erythema of the hands and soles of feet. Other features vary from renal involvement with glomerulonephritis to high blood pressure. Myocarditis, carditis, pleural effusion and pericardial effusion are other features of presentation. CNS involvement includes confusion and seizures, with focal neurological deficit, which makes the diagnosis of SLE very difficult in some cases. Aseptic bone necrosis, loss of visual fields, lymphadenopathy and gangrene of the fingers or toes is a bizarre presentation of this disease. Blood disorders like haemolytic anaemia (DCT positive) and thrombocytopenia with lymphopenia can also be manifested.

Autoantibodies are positive, including ANA and anti-double-strand DNA, which is more significant than any other autoantibody in diagnosing SLE. The C3 and C4 levels are low and indicate renal involvement. Corticosteroids can be given at a dose of 1–2 mg/kg/d with analgesia for pain relief. Other drugs can be added, if there is no response, such as azathioprine, and cyclophosphamide for children with proven renal involvement. The prognosis is not clear, but in general children do better than adults.

Case 2

1. c   Renal and Doppler ultrasound
   b   INR
   d   U&Es
   f   FBC
2. f   Right renal vein thrombosis
3. Rehydration
   Heparin
   Regular check of area and electrolytes

Right renal vein thrombosis

In acute renal failure, renal vein thrombosis should be ruled out, especially in neonates of a diabetic mother, one with HIE, or who is polyrhythmic and dehydrated. This is also true for children with cyanotic heart disease or septicaemia. The kidneys will be enlarged, there will be gross haematuria, oliguria with a low platelet count and a fall in haematocrit. The renal function will be abnormal on a DMSA scan and there will be no uptake of isotopes. Treatment is usually supportive, which includes peritoneal dialysis, if necessary to correct congestive heart failure, electrolyte imbalance, and intractable acidosis in cases of bilateral involvement. Heparin can be used in severe cases, but its use in mild cases is still controversial.

Case 3

1. c   Right and left knee X-ray
2. a   Guillain–Barré syndrome
    c   Myositis
    f   Hemiplegia (stroke)
3. Perventricular density on left
4. CK
    LP
    Increased white matter signals around anterior hornes of lateral ventricles on left and right
5. ADEM

Demyelination

Myelination in newborns is not formed until later in infancy. Demyelinating diseases in newborns are very difficult to diagnose until the end of the first year of life. The MRI scan is very good for picking up changes in white matter. There are few demyelinating diseases of childhood. A number of conditions affect the brain with demyelination, including ADEM, MS, and leukodystrophy. Transverse myelitis and Guillain–Barré (GB) syndrome affect the spinal cord.

ADEM is a version of MS in children. It is usually preceded by a viral-like illness, and symptoms can then appear as falls, hemiplegia and progressive limb weakness without sensory involvement. Cranial nerves can be involved earlier or later. The upper motor neuron signs are present in the early stages and bulbar palsy is common. Children may need protection of their airways at an early stage. Full testing, which includes neuroimaging and neurophysiology, is important as well as LP. A high dosage of i.v. steroids (methylprednisolone for 3–6 d) followed by oral corticosteroids for 6 weeks, withdrawn slowly, is the treatment of choice. There is no place for IVIG or plasmapheresis. The prognosis is good initially if there is no family history of MS. Children need to be followed up regularly, and neuroimaging can be carried out every 3–4 years if there are no symptoms.

MS is usually a disease of young adults, and children can be affected as early as 2 years of age. Presentation usually follows viral infection with ataxia, but other features may appear, such as encephalopathy, hemiplegia, or even seizures. Diagnosis can be made by recurrence of these symptoms with other features such as intraocular ophthalmoplegia, which affects one-third of children. The symptoms appear very quickly and remain for weeks or months, and then disappear with full or partial recovery. Children are usually lethargic, and limb ataxia and brisk tendon reflexes are a common finding. MRI is very good at picking up low signals in white matter, and contrasted CT may also be very helpful if MRI is not available. The prognosis is unpredictable and a course of corticosteroids may help.

Case 4

1. c   Endomyseal antibodies
   b   Upper GIT endoscopy with biopsy
   h   Ig and IgG subclass level
2. b   Total villous atrophy
   a   Lymphocyte infiltration
3. Gluten-sensitive enteropathy (coeliac disease)

Gluten-sensitive enteropathy (coeliac disease)

There are many causes of mouth ulcers, which include idiopathic causes, trauma, viral infection, inflammatory bowel disease, coeliac disease, and gastric ulcers.

The presentation of coeliac disease can be at any time of life but most usually during introduction of solids in the first year of life. There is usually one other member of the family affected and a detailed history is very important. The presentation is varied, from failure to thrive (FTT) in the early days to recurrent mouth ulcers and passing a lot of wind with anaemia. It is usually associated with malabsorption, in a form of anaemia and stool loss from time to time. Testing for antigliadin antibodies as well as endomyseal antibodies is part of the screen in children, with FTT in the first or second year of life. The presence of a high level of endomyseal antibodies indicates a very high suspicion of coeliac disease. The diagnosis can be confirmed by jejunual biopsy during illness or after changing to a gluten-free diet. It is a life-long condition and patients should be on a gluten-free diet, as the risk of intestinal lymphoma increases in people who do not adhere to this. Another complication associated with coeliac disease is occipital lobe calcification; whether this has any implications on epilepsy is still not very well recognised. A biopsy will show complete villous atrophy with lymphocytic infiltration and depth crypts. The other condition that may cause complete villous atrophy is tropical sprue. Partial villous atrophy is associated with CMPI and giardiasis.

Case 5

1. b   Hyperinflation
   c   Increased bronchial airway thickening
2. Compensated respiratory acidosis
3. b   NPA

Bronchiolitis

Bronchiolitis is one of the illnesses that affects infants and peaks between October to March each year. Some affected infants may need hospital admission and support, including expremature infants with CLD; those younger than 3 months of age; and infants with heart, lung, and CNS diseases. Between 1% and 2% may require admission to the PICU but the majority of bronchiolitic infants do not come to hospital. There is no vaccine but monoclonal antibodies given as i.m. injections for 5 months starting in September each year for premature babies with CLD or infants with heart, lung and CNS diseases reduce the risk of getting RSV bronchiolitis as well as the risk of admission to the PICU. Supportive treatment for infants admitted to hospital is required in the form of feeding, oxygen and care. Bronchodilators have no major role in treatment but there is no harm in trying them. Cross-infection is common, and hygiene as well as handwashing are vital to prevent this. NPA is not needed if the condition is clinically indicated to be RSV bronchiolitis but must be done for infants with CLD or heart problems, or those with an immunodeficiency problem.

Case 6

1. a   Congenital myotonic dystrophy
2. b   EMG
   a   Tensilon test
   d   Muscle biopsy
3. Poor
4. Supportive
   Genetic counselling
   Palliative care

Myotonic dystrophy

This is characterised by the association of myotonia with a dystrophic process of muscles with various endocrine and musculoskeletal abnormalities. It is transmitted as an autosomal dominant disorder and if present in the neonatal period is always transmitted from the mother but, in the adolescent period it is usually transmitted from the father. There is an expansion of a CTG triplet repeat associated with the gene for myotonia protein kinase. The length of the repeat usually increases in successive generations, especially when it is maternally transmitted. There is a strong relation between the length of the repeat and clinical severity and age of onset. The clinical presentation is variable, from generalised myotonia to prominent weakness. Myotonia can be seen by tapping the thenar muscle or tongue; the thumb will remain opposed and the tongue will remain dimpled. Relaxation of myotonia can be demonstrated by shaking hands with patients. Atrophy begins on the face and is followed by the shoulder girdle and leg muscles. Smooth-muscle involvement may be seen as decreased gastrointestinal motility, and constipation is a well-recognised feature. In adult patients there may be baldness, IDDM, cardiac myopathy, testicular atrophy, and peripheral nerve involvement. Intellectual impairment is very rare. The congenital form of myotonic dystrophy will usually start during the prenatal period with hydramnios, SGA, hypotonia, weakness, and arthrogryposis with joint contractures. The baby then becomes ventilator-dependent and dies within the first year of life. Myotonia is never observed before 3–4 years of age. Babies who survive the neonatal period are often mentally impaired, with bilateral ventricular dilatation and macrocephaly.

EMG is very helpful for children above the age of 5 years, but diagnosis can be made by clinical as well as by genetic study. Clinically, diagnosis can be made by shaking the mother's hand. Prenatal diagnosis can be made by chronic villi biopsy to look for the mytonic dystrophy gene. There is no truly effective treatment, but nifedipine can sometimes be helpful.

Case 7

1.   a   Brain, MRI
         b   EMG
         c   Urine toxicology
2.   a   Leptosirosis
         b   Myositis
         c   Drug abuse

Muscle spasms

Muscle pain following exercise is usually secondary to loss of fluids and electrolytes. Stretching may reverse the muscle spasms. Other spasms that are not related to exercise may be due to various causes: electrolyte imbalance, hypothyroidism, hyperthyroidism and hypoadrenalism are the main causes. Infection such as tetanus, which is very rare, leptospirosis, and strychnine poisoning may also cause muscle spasms but are rare causes. The metabolic causes are many and this can be diagnosed by measuring lactate, NH_4, and creatinine kinase, and any abnormalities of these should help in reaching the diagnosis. Muscle biopsy and EMG are very important in reaching the final diagnosis.

Pain management secondary to muscle spasms can be very difficult in children. Unresponsiveness to appropriate use of analgesic agents might be in addition to physical or psychological dimensions of the pain that are not addressed by the analgesics. In addition to appropriate analgesic therapy, the psychological needs of the child should be addressed directly and appropriate adjunctive physical modalities employed. Benzodiazepines can be used; even if they do not provide direct analgesic effects, they can reduce the distress associated with acute pain states by decreasing anxiety, insomnia, and muscle spasms that can be associated with acute pain.

Muscle spasms can present as seizures or a jumpy baby in the neonatal or infantile period. This is called hyperkeplexia and it begins with generalized hypertonicity accompanied by brisk muscle stretch reflexes, intermittent clonus, and an exaggerated startle response and it is benign. Anticonvulsant drugs will not be very helpful. Spasms can be familial or sporadic. Nose tapping in infants of affected families induced a uniform reaction of facial twitching accompanied by head extension, and a generalized flexor spasm, all of which may be a hallmark of hyperkeplexia. Small doses of benzodiazepines will almost always show some benefit; all affected individuals becoming asymptomatic by 2 years of age. There is no need for further investigations if a positive family history is suspected.

Case 8

1. d   Bartter syndrome
2.   Serum K, Na

Bartter's syndrome is a familial disorder characterised by activation of the renin–angiotensin–aldosterone pathway in an attempt to recover sodium chloride from the distal nephron. This causes an increase in potassium and hydrogen in urine secretion which will lead to hypokalaemic alkalosis. Affected individuals usually present with FTT, poor tone and lethargy, poor feeding, polydipsia and polyuria. It may also be associated with developmental delay. Hypercalciuria and bone demineralisation are due to an increased production of prostaglandin. Nephrocalcinosis is a serious and early complication. Potassium, sodium and chloride supplementation is needed as well as regular renal scans. Prostaglandin inhibitors such as indomethacin are indicated and angiotensin-converting enzyme (ACE) inhibitors (captopril) will help. If older children present with this syndrome, it is usually milder and they have no renal problem.

Case 9

1. d   IgG subclass
2. a   Prophylactic antibiotics
    d   Grommet insertion
    h   Regular inhaled corticosteroids for his asthma

Immune deficiency in children

Children with frequent severe bacterial or viral illnesses and required admissions should be treated with a high degree of suspicion for an immune deficiency problem, which could be primary or secondary. Repeated lung pneumonia affecting only one lobe or segment may indicate an anatomical problem. Multiorgan infection with different organisms may indicate an immune deficiency problem. Cases of IgG subclass G1–G3 deficiency usually present more frequently with a URTI or lung infection. Many affected people live normal lives. It is commonly associated with IgA deficiency, and any quantitative IgG subclass measurement should be interpreted in conjunction with antibody response and a clinical scenario. In symptomatic children, prophylactic co-trimoxazole may be needed over the winter. Only a small of group of children who have a failed antibody response to immunisation with IgG subclass deficiency require regular i.v. immunoglobulin every 4–6 weeks. During the winter, the start of school and after school breaks, children may be more vulnerable to viral infections. Some may have up to 6–8 URTIs per year; this occurs most often between the ages of 3–7 years. This is not an immune deficiency problem and testing of the immune system should only be undertaken to reassure parents and doctors, which usually is not needed.

Case 10

1. a   Streptococcal throat infection
    e   Crohn's disease
    b   Coxsackie virus A infection
2. f   ASO titres
    c   Throat swab

Streptococcal throat infection

Among the causes of mouth ulcers are streptococcal infections as well as viral infections. There are different groups of streptococcal throat infections. Beta-haemolytic streptococci is the commonest and group A are more so than group B. A throat swab is important to confirm the infection. A throat swab that includes swabbing the tonsillar and posterior pharynx is essential. Latex agglutination and enzyme-linked immunoassay are rapid test's developed recently, which can be done within 15–30 min on a throat swab to diagnose Group A streptococcal antigen. Treatment can then be started. Treating red throats is always a problem. Most throat redness is due to viral infection. Large, inflamed, tonsils are indicative of antibiotic use if the child is unwell, but if the child is well, a throat swab should be carried out promptly and treatment can be given when it is ready, after 24–48 hours. If the culture is positive for group A beta-haemolytic streptococcal infection, then penicillin V for 10 days is recommended to eradicate the infection completely. Compliance is always a problem, but advice to finish the course as well as to repeat the throat swab is preferable. The tender rash on the lower limbs is erythema nodosum.

Case 11

For the last 4 weeks, a boy aged 11 years has been seen in an outpatient department with a history of cough and abdominal pain. He is passing frequent stools, sometimes containing mucus. His appetite is not very good and he has lost some weight. One of his schoolteachers describes him as having lost his touch and become very nervous. His father died when the boy was 9 years old, following a cerebral haemorrhage. His sister is 16 years old and is doing very well. His mother was admitted to hospital 1 year ago with a possible diagnosis of breast cancer. Later that year, all of his mother's results came back as normal.

The cough is described as dry, mainly occurring at night, and there are no other symptoms. There is no history of travel abroad since his father's death and he is a youth member of a local football club. The family lives in a three-bedroomed detached house and his mother works as a sales manager, full time in the last 6 months.

He is very anxious and is talking with a low voice, as he had an accident in his underwear today, while he was playing football. His abdomen is soft, with mild tenderness in the right iliac fossa and his chest is clear.

ESR	70 mm/hour
Hb	11 g/dl
MCV	77 fl
PLT	$500 \times 10^9/l$
LFT	Normal

1. What is the most useful bedside examination that can be carried out?
   a Blood pressure
   b Urine dipstick
   c Fundoscopy
   d OFC
   e Height and weight
   f Blood glucose by multisticks test
   g Rectal examination

He was admitted overnight and was coughing most of the night. All other observations are normal. There is a small mark on his bed, which looks like mucus with blood.

2. What else can be done?
   a Stool for culture
   b Upper and lower GIT endoscopy with biopsies
   c Barium swallow
   d Stool for occult blood
   e Perineal examination
   f Abdominal MRI

       g   Check child-protection register
       h   Arrange for forensic medical examination (FME)
3.   What are the three abnormalities visible on this slide?

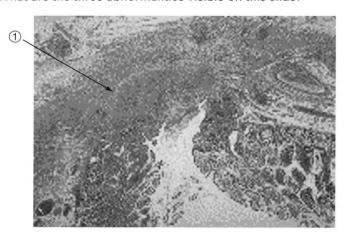

       a   Lymphocyte infiltration
       b   Goblet cells
       c   Non-caseating granulomatous changes
       d   Crypt abscess
       d   Ulcers
       e   Giant cells
       f   Transmural inflammation
4.   What is the most likely diagnosis?
       a   Crohn's disease
       b   Ulcerative colitis
       c   Eosinophilic colitis
       d   Schwachman syndrome
       e   Cystic fibrosis (CF)
       f   GIT tuberculosis
       g   Recto-anal fistula
       h   Child sexual abuse (CSA)

Case 12

A 20-month-old child presented with a sudden onset of a dropped right upper eyelid. There is no other abnormality. There is a history of recent hand–foot–mouth disease, which occurred just 1 week earlier. The family were camping in a forest for 2 nights, 6 weeks ago. Her brother, who is 10 years old, complained of a headache 1 year ago, which resolved after a few months. The mother has suffered from cluster migraine but not in the last 6 years. Her father is a milkman and is dyslexic. Her two older sisters are fit and well and there are no pets in the house.

In an eye examination, a dropped right upper eyelid was noted, with a fixed and dilated pupil. She is having difficulty with right eye movement, especially while looking down and to the side. There is no facial asymmetry. The other cranial nerves are intact. Her tone, power, reflexes and gait are normal. CT and MRI brain scans were reported as normal.

1. What is the diagnosis?
   a   Myasthenia gravis
   b   Eye myoclonia
   c   Fourth nerve palsy
   d   Third nerve palsy
   e   Optic neuritis
   f   Cervical rib
   g   Intraocular ophthalmoplegia
2. List three possible common causes
   a   Idiopathic
   b   Benign increased intracranial pressure (BICH)
   c   *Mycoplasma* infection
   d   *Borrelia* infection (Lyme disease)
   e   SLE
   f   Trauma
3. What are the next three investigations and one bedside test that should be carried out?
   a   Fundi examination
   b   *Borrelia* antibodies
   c   ANA
   d   *Mycoplasma* titres
   e   Blood film
   f   Mantoux test
   g   CXR
   h   Blood pressure
   i   Visual field examination
   j   Urine dipstick for protein
   k   Check weight and height

Case 13

A 4-year-old girl presented with a sudden onset of left-sided hemiplegia. She has been unwell for 2 days, with headache, tiredness and lethargy. There is no history of recent infection. She was diagnosed as having a heart murmur, but no structural abnormalities have been found following ECHO and 24-hour ECG. A venous hum was diagnosed.

A year ago her mother had a cardiac arrest preceded by severe headache. She was in a vegetative state with coma and massive brain damage. She used to suffer from migraine throughout her life. The girl's test results are:

On examination Left hemiparesis with left facial weakness.
CRP   20
ESR   50 mm/hour

LP	Normal, including serology and oligoclonal band
Clotting/FBC	Normal
LFT and NH_4, blood gases, urine AAs and organic acids	
Lactate	Normal
(both CSF and blood)	Normal
MRI/MRA	Show right ganglia infarction with evidence of right posterior artery reducing calliper

1. List four possible causes
2. List four important investigations

Case 14

A 3-month-old infant presented with a history of increasing frequency of stool, up to 10 times/day for the last 3 weeks. The stool is runny and contains mucus most of the time. On one occasion it was mixed with blood. His weight 3 weeks ago was 5.2 kg and it is now 5.020 kg. He is feeding very well, every 4 hours on the breast, and his mother had been told not to give him any dairy products for 2 weeks. After this treatment, there was still no improvement. He has a runny nose and there is no evidence of chesty cough or discomfort. There is no evidence of soreness on his bottom. He is the only child of a young Caucasian couple, with no family history of illness. He was born at term and had no neonatal problems.

On examination, he looks happy and is smiling, with scratch marks on his forehead. He has no rash on his body. His abdomen is soft and his chest is clear. His face resembles his mother's, with an anxious look. The test results are:

Hb	12.5 g/dl
WCCs	$8.6 \times 10^9/l$ (N 60%, L 38%, E 0.4%)
PLT	$160 \times 10^9/l$
Alb	39 g/l
Total protein	65g/l
Alk. Ph	234 mmol/l
Stool $\times 3$	No growth after 5 days
CRP	0.5
ESR	10 mm/hour
Stool for reducing substances	Negative

1. What other three investigations should be carried out?
    a   Stool pH
    b   Hydrogen breath test
    c   Lactose quantitative in stool
    d   Endoscopy and biopsy
    e   Blood film

f   Stool for fat
g   Sweat test
h   Ig and IgG subclass
i   Coeliac screen
j   Skin test
2. What is the most likely diagnosis?
a   Lactose milk intolerance
b   Colitis
c   Infection
d   Food allergy
e   CF
f   Congenital enteropathy
3. What four steps should you take to manage this infant?
a   Prednisolone for 3 weeks
b   Azathioprine
c   Hydrolysed milk products
d   Lactose-free milk
e   Creon
f   Weekly weight
g   Re-challenge with lactose and biopsy

Case 15

A 3-hour-old baby was found by a midwife to be cyanosed; she called the paediatrician. The cyanosis started as soon as the baby started feeding but there was no apnoea. His Sat in air is 66% and on 100% was 77%. He was born at term and a neonatal scan at the booking-in appointment was reported as normal. His mother used to drink alcohol but stopped as soon as she knew she was pregnant. She smokes between 5 and 10 cigarettes/d and does not use drugs. She is hepatitis C-positive and her two other children are healthy. She is hepatitis B- and HIV-negative. The hyperoxic test was carried out on the baby but the Sat was still in the high 70s. His BP is 70/40 mmHg, with a mean of 45 mmHg from the umbilical artery catheter (UAC). Pulses are difficult to feel, even after resuscitation. He was intubated and ventilated before transfer to a specialist cardiac centre. He is acidotic, on arterial blood gas with a PCV of 60 fl. The CXR shows a haziness of the perihilar area. There is no murmur but the first heart sound is faint. An i.v. antibiotic was started and a cranial US was reported as normal.

1. What needs to be done immediately?
a   Exchange transfusion
b   CXR
c   Arterial line
d   Peripheral line
e   Start prostaglandin infusion
f   Half-correction of acidosis by bicarbonate
g   Arrange transfer to specialist centre
h   Start i.v. antibiotics (cephalosporins)
i   Restrict the fluid to 40% of requirement

    j   Sedation with morphine
    k   Start i.v. dopamine infusion 5 µg/kg/min

He was treated and 2 weeks later had an aortography to help in diagnosing and planning corrective surgery for his condition after echocardiography.

2.   What is the abnormality on this X-ray

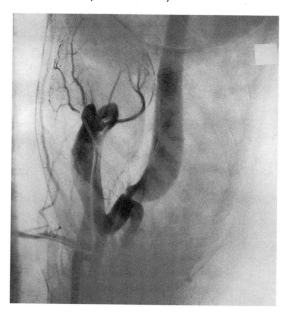

3.   Which three conditions are associated with this problem?
    a   Marfan syndrome
    b   Noonan syndrome
    c   Turner syndrome
    d   DiGeorge syndrome
    e   Fetal alcohol syndrome
    f   William syndrome
    g   Down syndrome

Case 16

A GP referred a 3-year-old girl with a history of possible seizures. She goes to bed and 3 hours later, she wakes up, looks frightened and says, 'The white man coming and the white man going'. Then she starts reaching for objects and repeats this many times. Her eyes are sometimes open but most of the time they are closed. This pattern is repeated up to ten times each night for 3–4 nights per week. She has never had jerks or shaking events. She is one of four children, who are well and living with their mother, as their father left home 1 year ago. She still sleeps 1–2 hours during the daytime. Her development is compatible with her age and she has been described as a 'hyperactive girl' by her mother.

The mother is quite anxious as the girl's uncle on her mother's side suffers from epilepsy. A general and systemic examination reveals no abnormalities and the awake EEG shows no abnormality. The FBC, Mg, Ca, Glu, and LFT tests are all normal. She was treated with sodium valproate up to 40 mg/kg/d, but she is still having the same problem and is now starting to wet herself during the daytime.

1.   What is the diagnosis?
   a   Nightmares
   b   Generalised seizures
   c   Complex partial seizures
   d   Sleep disorder
   e   Hallucination
   f   Behaviour problem
   g   Benign Rolandic epilepsy of childhood
   h   Landau–Kleffner syndrome
2.   Which three other investigations should be carried out, and in what order?
   a   Cranial MRI
   b   Cranial CT
   c   Sleep EEG
   d   Video telemetry
   e   Ambulatory EEG
   f   ECG
   g   Partial metabolic screen
   h   Urine toxicology

Her asleep EEG shows some paroxysmal slow waves arising anteriorly.

3.   What is the drug of choice that should be added to control her seizures?
   a   Sodium valproate
   b   Carbamazepine
   c   Lamotrigine
   d   Vigabatrin
   e   Topiramate
   f   Steroids
   g   Tiagabine
   h   Levatricetam

Case 17

An 8-year-old girl was admitted to hospital with rectal bleeding. This was described as 'fresh blood' on several occasions in the past and always after emptying her bowel. She was treated for constipation, and her lower GIT colonscopy, carried out locally by an adult physician, was normal. She is not complaining of any abdominal pain or other symptoms. Her mother says she has become weaker and weaker in the last 3 months. The girl has lost some weight and looks pale. Her father was diagnosed as having pulmonary tuberculosis 7 years go and was treated successfully. Systemic and general examinations show no abnormalities. The perineal region is clear and there is no evidence of an anal fissure or old scars. Other test results are:

Hb	7.2 g/dl
WCC	$6.7 \times 10^9/l$
PLT	$450 \times 10^9/l$
ESR	25 mm/hour
INR	1.5
PT, APTT	Normal ranges
LFT, U&Es	Normal ranges
Stool	No growth after 5 days
AXR/US	Normal
Mantoux test	Negative with 1:10 000 and 1:1000

1. What are the 3 most likely diagnoses?
    a   Intestinal polyps
    b   Inflammatory bowel disease
    c   Infective gastroenteritis
    d   Constipation
    e   Meckel's diverticulum
    f   Intestinal tuberculosis
    g   Duodenal ulcers
    h   Haemorrhoids
    i   Child sexual abuse
    j   Anal fissure
2. What abnormalities appear on this X-ray film?

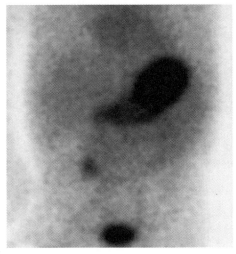

3. What is the diagnosis?

Case 18

A 6-month-old infant presented with jaundice and FTT. He was born at term and there were no neonatal problems. He is breast-fed and is now on solids. He is taking his food without difficulty. At the age of 5 months, he was seen by GPs, when a history of cough and a heart murmur were diagnosed, and he was referred to hospital. Over the last 3 days he has become more lethargic, is not interested in his food, and his colour is changing.

His father has a valvular heart problem, but no surgery was required and there are no other siblings. There is an ejection systolic murmur on the left side of the chest, mainly loud at the second intercostal space. The liver is about 4 cm below the right costal margin, with yellow sclera. Stool colour is normal. His urine is described as 'dark' by his mother. His father has a long face and there are other abnormal features on the spinal X-rays (butterfly vertebrae).

Hb	11.5 g/dl
WWC	$11 \times 10^9/l$ (N 65%)
PLT	$320 \times 10^9/l$
Bilirubin	265 mmol/l (20% conjugated)
Alk. Ph	660 IU/l
ALT	120 IU/l
Alb	32 g/l
γGT	80 IU/l
CMV IgG	Positive
Caeruloplasmine	Normal
Hepatitis B,C,A serology	Negative
US of abdomen	Large liver with normal consistency and no splenomegaly

1. What are the two most useful investigations that should be carried out?
    a ECG
    b CXR
    c ECHO
    d Liver biopsy
    e Repeat viral serology
    f Bone marrow biopsy
    g Muscle biopsy
    h White cell enzyme
    i Urine for organic acids and GAGs
    j Blood for AAs
    k Urine toxicology
    l Transferrin level
2. What is the diagnosis?
    a Hurler syndrome
    b Hunter syndrome
    c Carbohydrate glycosylated protein deficiency syndrome
    d Alagille syndrome
    e Glycogen storage disease type 1b

      f   Chronic active hepatitis
      g   Pomp disease

Case 19

A mother brought her 10-year-old daughter, who has a history of frequent cough and a high temperature for the last 6 days. Her cough has been getting worse over the last year, in spite of asthma treatment and courses of antibiotics prescribed by her GP. The cough is productive and has been consistent for the last 2 days.

She was born full term, with no problems in the first 2 years. On her second birthday she contracted a URTI and was treated with antibiotics for 2 weeks, as her symptoms took a long time to clear. The family lives in a council flat and recently one child in her school was diagnosed as having pulmonary tuberculosis. The test results are:

Mantoux test	Negative with 1:10 000 and 1:1000
CRP	25
ESR	10 mm/hour and repeated after one week 12 mm/hour
WCC	$10 \times 10^9/l$ (L 40%, N 57%)
Sweat test	Weight 110 bg (Na 30 mmol)

1.   What are the abnormalities on this CXR?

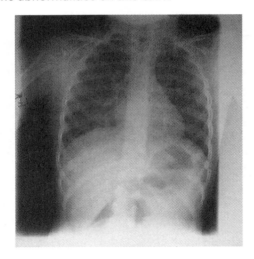

      a   Hyperinflated right lung
      b   Left upper lobe consolidation
      c   Tracheal stenosis
      d   Foreign body on right lower bronchial tree supplying lower segment lobe

  e   Cystic changes on right lower lobe
  f   Bronchial thickening
  g   Bilateral hilar shadows
  h   Right lower lobe segmental consolidation in two X-rays
2.   What are the next investigations that should be carried out in order?
  a   Bronchoscopy with lavage
  b   Bronchial lavage
  c   Cilia motility study
  d   Chest CT
  e   Lung biopsy
  f   Chest MRI scan
  g   Barium swallow
  h   Transoesophageal echocardiography
  i   DNA linkage study for CF
  j   Ig
  k   HIV antibody
  l   Skin allergy test
  m   Spirometry
3.   Which two therapeutic steps should be taken for this patient?
  a   Chest physiotherapy
  b   I.v. antibiotics
  c   Lobectomy
  d   Lung transplant
  e   IVIG every 4 weeks
  f   Regular chest scans
  g   Overnight continuous positive airway pressure (CPAP)
  h   Genetic counselling
4.   What is the most likely diagnosis?

Case 20

A baby was admitted to hospital with a history of apnoea and possible seizures. He was born at term after a prolonged second stage of labour. The Apgar score was 8 at 1 min and 9 at 5 min. Mother and baby were discharged home 6 hours later and a health visitor visited on two occasions. He is now 5 days old and breast-fed.

An hour after admission, the baby's Sat level dropped to 85% and the nurse noticed a twitching of his right leg and arm. This continued for about 10 min. The baby was transferred to a high-dependency bed and regular monitoring was carried out. Various blood tests were carried out and the baby was put on benzylpenicillin and gentamicin. LP revealed no abnormalities. The baby carried on fitting intermittently and he was given a loading dose of phenobarbitone and put on maintenance therapy.

The next morning he had another 3-minute seizure, affecting mainly the right side of his body. The test results are:

NH_4 28 mmol/l
Lactate   1.9 mmol/l

pH	7.35
PCO_2	4.2 kPa
HCO_3	21
BE	0.01
PO_2	8.3 kPa
INR	1.1
Hb	17 g/dl
PLT	$270 \times 10^9/l$
CRP	< 5
BS	4.5 mmol/l
Mg	0.92 mmol/l
Ca	2.45 mmol/l
MSSU	Negative
Urine toxicology	Negative
Blood C	Negative

1.   What is the next single investigation you should carry out?
    a   EEG
    b   Cranial US
    c   Cranial CT
    d   Metabolic screen
    e   Thrombophilia screen
    f   Skull X-ray
    g   Skeletal survey

He continued to have seizures once every hour for 3 hours of < 1 min in duration; after a half loading dose of phenobarbitone, he stopped fitting.

2.   What are three abnormalities on this cranial CT?

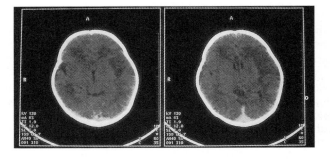

    a   Cerebral oedema
    b   Subarachnoid haemorrhage
    c   Subdural effusion
    d   Small lateral ventricles
    e   Dilated ventricles
    f   Attenuation and low density of left parietotemporal lobe
    g   Basal ganglia calcification

h   Brain atrophy
i   Shifting of midline
3. What is one single bedside clinical test that should be carried out earlier?
a   Measuring blood pressure
b   Fundi examination
c   Repeated BS
d   Measuring temperature
e   Oxygen Sat
f   ECG
g   Testing all reflexes
4. What are three possible causes?
a   Middle cerebral artery infarct
b   Birth trauma
c   Shaken baby syndrome
d   Intercerebral bleed
e   Hypoxic ischaemic encephalopathy (HIE)
f   Neonatal seizures
g   Accidental trauma

ANSWERS 11–20

Case 11

1. e   Weight and height
2. e   Perineal examination
   b   Upper and lower GIT endoscopy with biopsy
3. c   Non-caseating granulomatous changes
   e   Giant cells
   g   Transmural inflammation
4. a   Crohn's disease

Crohn's disease

This disease can involve any part of the GIT system. There is always a delay in diagnosis of this condition as presentation is not characteristic but a high index of suspicion is needed. Colicky abdominal pain and diarrhoea with or without growth failure are highly indicative of inflammatory bowel disease, and investigations should be initiated to find the cause. Blood will show iron deficiency anaemia with a high ESR and CRP in the acute recurrent phase. Thrombocytosis and hypoalbuminaemia may also be present and are indicative of active illness. An abdominal X-ray with barium may not be tolerated very well, but it will show skip lesions and narrowing of the lumen, thickening and fissuring of the bowel wall and fistula formation – all highly indicative of Crohn's disease. The MRI scan is also very useful and helpful in diagnosis if barium swallow or endoscopy cannot be carried out. A technetium-labelled leukocyte scan is proving useful in follow-up and diagnosis but is still in the early stages of development. The diagnostic procedure is upper or lower GIT endoscopy with biopsy. The inflammation is transmural, resulting in sinus tracts or fistula formation. The bowel mucosa may look inflamed, and small shallow, aphthoid or linear ulcers may be present. Deep fissures lead to a cobblestone appearance later on, as will structuring. The hallmark is the finding of non-caseating epithelioid granulomata with giant cells.

Case 12

1. d Third nerve palsy
2. a Idiopathic
   d Lyme disease
   b BICH
3. a Fundi examination
   b *Borrelia* antibodies
   e Blood film
   d *Mycoplasma* titres

Oculomotor nerve palsy (third nerve palsy)

Third nerve palsy can be isolated or associated with other nerve palsies, mainly of the abducens cranial nerve. It can be congenital and is usually unilateral and complete. Only half of affected patients can be diagnosed during the neonatal period. It can be familial or due to trauma of the orbit at birth. Most cases are idiopathic. The affected eye is exotropic and usually amblyopic. Brain tumours are among the many causes of increased cranial pressure and third nerve palsy. In general, compression of the oculomotor nerve by a herniated uncus produces only involvement of papillary fibres with unresponsive mydriasis. Complete paralysis of the third cranial nerve may result in ptosis and extrinsic ocular muscle deficit. An MRI scan of the brain is indicated to exclude the possibility of an intracranial mass. Dilated pupils will exclude myasthenia gravis, but an edrophonium chloride test is indicated if the pupils are normal. Cosmetic surgery is required, but will not improve ocular motility and visual function.

Case 13

1. Basilar artery migraine attack
   AV malformation
   Cerebral infarct
   Infection
2. Arterial angiography
   Protein levels
   DNA double strand
   Thrombophilic screen

Headaches in children

Types of headaches
Acute
Acute recurrent
Chronic progressive
Chronic non-progressive
Cluster headache
Epileptic headache
Psychogenic
Mixed

Acute headache may be due to migraine, cerebrovascular bleed, trauma, meningitis, encephalitis or drugs.

Migraine headache is a recurrent headache and is characterised by a positive family history, visual aura, nausea, unilateral pain (throbbing) and gastrointestinal symptoms. Other causes should be excluded.

The incidence of migraine in children is 1.2–3.2% at the age of 7 years, and 4–19% by the age of 15 years. It is more prevalent in females and has a genetic component. About 2.8 school days per year are lost as a result of migraine, and children commonly have migraine without an aura. Children do not usually have unilateral headache. The pathophysiology of headache can be explained as vasodilatation, vasoconstriction, oedema, and inflammation of the cerebral vessels, which can lead to pain. These are the most common pathophysiological changes associated with migraine as suggested by many neurologists.

The clinical features of migraine attack can be divided into phases. The prodrome phase is the first, and is associated with a change in mood or activity level. This is followed by an aura (this occurs in 10–50% of paediatric migraine attacks) consisting of photopsia, scotoma, numbness, tingling, ataxia, dizziness and vertigo. The next phase, headache, is mainly bilateral and classically not unilateral. The resolution phase usually follows the headache phase, which may last 1–4 hours. The postdrome phase occurs after the headache is resolved by sleep or analgesia. Patients will feel lethargic and anorexic and experience mood disturbances.

There are a number of types of migraine. Migraine with an aura is called 'classical migraine'. Migraine without an aura is called 'common migraine'. Complicated migraine is another form, and may present as hemiplegic migraine, ophthalmoplegic migraine, confusional migraine or basilar artery migraine. Atypical forms of migraine are less frequent than others, e.g. with cyclic vomiting, recurrent abdominal pain and hemiplegia.

Another type of headache is 'chronic progressive', which is characterised by a daily headache with an increase in severity and frequency. Intercranial pathology should be suspected. It usually does not respond to analgesia and may or may not be associated with neurological symptoms and signs. It may or may not be associated with behavioural problems and needs urgent investigation, including neuroimaging in most patients.

When seeing children with headache, a thorough clinical examination is very important and it is important to remember to examine the skin; chart weight, height and head circumference; listen for cranial bruits; measure blood pressure and carry out a detailed CNS and systemic examination (of the optic disc, eye movements, motor asymmetry, coordination and reflexes).

There are high-priority patients who may need urgent neuroimaging scans, including children with acute headache or chronic progressive headache with abnormal or focal neurological abnormalities, and papilloedema. Children with neurocutaneous syndromes (NF or TS) and headache also need urgent neuroimaging. It is very unusual in children < 3 years, and this is very significant. Other low-risk groups include those with chronic non-progressive headache, mixed headache, classic or common migraine, or a variation in headache location.

Indications for neuroimaging in 78 paediatric patients with headaches. Maytal et al. *Ped.* 1995; **96**:413–417

Headache onset at younger age (< 5 years)	4
Increasing severity or frequency of headache	5
Abnormalities on ocular or neurological examination	6
Headache provoked by changing position of head	2
Focal symptoms or signs during headaches	7
Systemic symptoms, e.g. weight loss, fatigue	11
Doctors' and parents' concern about cerebral mass	12
Not specified	12
Atypical headache pattern	12

Drugs that are helpful in the treatment of headache are paracetamol, ibuprofen, codeine phosphate, ergot derivatives (to be avoided in children), propranolol and clonidine. Other drugs that may be used if one or a combination of two of the above-mentioned drugs are not controlling headache include phenytoin and phenobarbitone, carbamazepine, gabapentin, sodium valproate and lamotrigine, calcium-channel blockers (nifedipine, cyproheptadine, flunarizine). Triptans ($5HT_{1B\ 1D}$ recepter agonists (e.g. sumatriptan) are very effective in aborting migraine attack and can be used in children aged 16 and older. Use in children at younger ages is not yet licensed and will be left to the individual specialist to decide.

Anti-emetics that may be used in the treatment of nausea and vomiting accompanying childhood migraine are promethazine (Phenergan), trimethobenzamide (Tigan), prochlorperazine, metoclopramide, and hydroxyzine.

Case 14

1. b   Hydrogen breath test
   c   Lactose quantitative study
   d   Endoscopy and biopsy
2. a   Lactose milk intolerance
   b   Colitis
3. c   Hydrolysed milk products
   d   Lactose-free milk
   f   Weekly weight measurement
   g   Re-challenge with lactose and biopsy

Congenital enteropathy (dietary intolerance)

Dietary intolerance can present as vomiting and/or diarrhoea in the
first few weeks of life. Lactose intolerance usually presents with
diarrhoea. Lactose intolerance secondary to gastroenteritis is not
common in the early days of life. Reducing substances will be a
positive step in the infant with diarrhoea. Primary lactose
intolerance will cause diarrhoea but it is not a common condition.
These infants usually present with diarrhoea and failure to thrive
(FTT). Weight loss is common but rarely associated with vomiting.
The blood results will be normal apart from signs of dehydration and
acidosis. Reducing substances will be positive, but a definitive
diagnosis can be made by small intestinal biopsy. A hydrogen breath
test will be helpful, but it is difficult to perform in small babies.
Lactose-free milk should be prescribed for babies with primary or
secondary lactose intolerance. Secondary lactose intolerance will
resolve and cows' milk should be tried for 3–6 months. Primary
lactose intolerance is a life-long condition but is not severe in later life
with cow's milk.

Glucose or galactose malabsorption, congenital chlorodiarrhoea,
abetalipoproteinaemia, acrodermatitis enteropathica, and
congenital microvillous atrophy are other forms of congenital
enteropathy. Cows' milk protein intolerance is another form of
enteropathy that may follow gastroenteritis and can
present either with vomiting as allergy or has diarrhoea as
enteropathy. The mucosa will be flat and recovery can be achieved by
changing to whey soya milk; challenge with cows' milk should be
made after 3–6 months.

Case 15

1. e   Start prostaglandin infusion
   f   Half correction of acidosis by bicarbonate
   g   Arrange transfer to specialist centre
2. Postductal aortic stenosis
3. c   Turner syndrome
   e   Fetal alcohol syndrome
   g   Down syndrome

Coarctation of the aorta

There are two types of coarctaton of the aorta: preductal (infantile) and posductal (adult). They cause a narrowing of the aortic arch between the left subclavian origin and ductus arteriosus. The aortic valve is usually bicuspid. The pulmonary venous and arterial pressure will be raised as a consequence of obstruction to aortic blood flow, or of a left-to-right shunt with patent ductus arteriosus or VSD. The rise in systemic blood pressure is due to mechanical obstruction, and increased renin production is due to reduced renal perfusion. Coarctation can present at any time within the first month of life. In the first few hours of life the commonest presentation is shock and a respiratory problem, which may be related to ductus arteriosus closure. Weak or absent femoral pulses with a wide gap between the blood pressure of the upper and lower limbs is an indicator of possible left ventricular outlet obstruction, mainly coarctation. The second heart sound, which will be loud, with no murmur most of the time, and a strong apex beat due to ventricular hypertrophy, are other features that may aid the clinical diagnosis. The child is acidotic, and ventilatory support is required as well as keeping the duct open by prostaglandin infusion. Antibiotic cover should also be started, as well as correction of acidosis with fluid and bicarbonate. The team of specialists should be informed and arrangements for transfer should start. If the duct is closed and the baby is getting worse, then a septostomy can be performed under ECHO guidance by a well-trained cardiologist.

Early CXR may show pulmonary oedema and cardiomegaly, and appearance of a 'Swiss loaf' heart can be seen. Rib notching occurs in older children who become symptomatic later. An ECG in newborn babies will show right ventricular hypertrophy. Echocardiography is diagnostic and the pressure gradient across the obstruction can be estimated. Cardiac catheterisation and angiography should preferably not be carried out in sick children, but can be done if the diagnosis is uncertain. Surgical correction and balloon dilatation angioplasty can be used, and balloon dilatation is effective in older children or in recoarctation after surgery.

Case 16

1. a   Complex partial seizures
2. c   Sleep EEG
    a   Cranial MRI
    f   ECG
3. b   carbamazepine

Temporal lobe epilepsy

This is the most common cause of complex partial seizures in children and adults. It is usually preceded by an aura (hallucination and illusion, epigastric sensation in young children with fear, head deviation and posturing in children < 2 years of age). The seizure may start as staring or behaviour arrest and then be followed by automatism (lip smacking, licking, chewing or swallowing movements). Some other bizarre behaviour such as fingering or fumbling with clothes is also frequent and can be misleading in the diagnosis of this condition. Tonic posturing and head rotation are often seen in those < 2 years old during their usual seizures; sometimes there is just jerking or twitching of one side of the body which may or may not be followed by generalised tonic–clonic seizure. This will last 1–2 min and be followed by confusion and/or intense tiredness. In older children and adolescents, mesial temporal lobe epilepsy may be present.

Mesial temporal lobe epilepsy

This is characterised histologically by atrophy and gliosis of the hippocampus, and often the amygdala. It is associated with long unilateral febrile seizures in 40–60% of cases, and partial seizures start in the first 10 years of life. Seizures are marked by behavioural arrest, staring, automatism (facial), and dystonic posturing of the arm contralateral to the discharging temporal lobe while automatism occurs in the ipsilateral arm.

EEG
There is an interictal anterior temporal spike focus or sometimes a paroxysmal theta rhythm. An ictal EEG will show a diffuse discharge on the other side. Cranial MRI using an epilepsy protocol will help to identify areas of abnormality in the hippocampus or temporal lobe. In some cases in which surgery is required and the focus of discharge could not be determined, a PET scan or ictal and interictal SECT scan may help to localise the focus of the discharge. Many cases have been operated on with temporal lobectomy, and the outcome has been very good.

Case 17

1. a Intestinal polyps
   e Meckel's diverticulum
   j Anal fissue
2. Increased uptake
3. Meckel's diverticulum

Meckel's diverticulum

This arises from the vitellointestinal duct, which leads from the primitive gut to the yolk sac. It occurs in 2% of the population (2 in. long and 2 ft. from the ileocaecal valve). The vitellointestinal duct may cause other abnormalities. If it remains open, this will lead to fistulae, or a fibrous cord from the umbilicus to the ileum may act as an axis for localised volvulus or lead to bowel obstruction. Meckel's diverticulum may become inflamed and cause bleeding or intussusception, or may present as acute appendicitis. It usually

contains heterotropic gastric mucosa, which is the main cause of
bleeding. This is usually a painless bleeding in preschool children. It
is usually a large haemorrhage with passage of bright maroon blood.
Meckel's scan is helpful in diagnosis by ^{99m}Tcpertechnetate isotope
scan, which has an affinity for parietal cells. Diverticulectomy is the
treatment and there is no recurrence.

Case 18

1. c   Echocardiography
    d   Liver biopsy
2. Alagille syndrome

Intrahepatic biliary hypoplasia (Alagille syndrome)

This is usually inherited as an autosomal dominant syndrome.
Most cases have jaundice from the neonatal period which disappears
by childhood or adult life; sometimes it can present as pruritis
only. The longstanding cholestasis causes pruritis, jaundice,
hypercholesterolaemia and xanthelasma. One-quarter of patients will
have cardiac abnormalities, affecting mainly peripheral pulmonary
artery stenosis. There are atypical phenotypic features, which include
hypertelorism, a pointed nose, deep-set eyes, overhanging forehead
and a straight nose with a small pointed chin. A high serum
cholesterol level will support the diagnosis. There is cirrhosis of the
liver in 15% of cases and other liver disease in 10%. Treating pruritis,
hypercholesterolaemia and cholestasis helps to prevent further
complications in these patients. Cardiac surgery is not always
indicated but regular follow-up with echocardiography is vital.
Genetic counselling is important and prenatal diagnosis has not yet
been established.

Case 19

1. a   Hyperinflated right lung
    h   Right lower lobe segmental consolidation in two X-rays
2. d   Chest CT
    a   Bronchoscopy with lavage
    i   DNA linkage study for CF
    j   Ig
3. I.v. antibiotics for acute infection for 2 weeks
    Chest physiotherapy
4. Bronchiectasis

Bronchiectasis

This is a chronic lung diseases that can follow infection and especially
pulmonary tuberculosis, which has started to appear more frequently
in recent years. It is usually associated with congenital lung
abnormalities such as bronchomalacia, sequestration, aspiration of a
foreign body that is missed, and chronic chest infection associated

with CF, ciliary dyskinesia, or primary immune deficiency. The usual symptoms are cough, wheeze, poor weight gain, bad breath, purulent sputum and recurrent chest infection. Finger clubbing is another feature; it can be easily tested by demonstrating diamond signs (putting fingernails of thumbs apposite to each other the diamond sign will disappear), or looking at the curvature of the nails or testing fluid in nail buds. Chest X-ray may show an area of consolidation, usually one of the lower lobe segments, but chest CT is very helpful, and will show the area of consolidation as well as the dilated bronchioles. Bronchoscopy will be helpful if the presence of a foreign body or any congenital bronchial or alveolar abnormalities are suspected. A lung function study will help to see if the patient suffers from an obstructive or restrictive lung problem. Physiotherapy and bronchodilators will help, but intermittent antibiotics when sputum shows infection are important to prevent further damage. Surgical intervention is not necessary if the patient is followed up closely and antibiotics are given when needed.

Case 20

1. c   Cranial CT
2. f   Attenuation and low density of left parietotemporal lobe
   a   Cerebral oedema
   d   Small lateral ventricles
3. b   Fundi examination
4. a   A right middle cerebral artery infarct
   c   Shaken baby syndrome
   g   Accidental trauma

Neonatal cerebrovascular accident

This is more common in full-term than preterm babies. Neonatal infarction can be divided into three types: (1) Single-artery infarction, which may be caused by injury to the cervical portion of the carotid artery during difficult delivery; but this is very rare and most of the time a cause cannot be found; (2) Multi-artery infarction may be caused by congenital heart disease and less frequently by perinatal distress or disseminated intravascular coagulation and polycythaemia; (3) Arterial border zone infarction (insula) may be caused during active resuscitation as a consequence of hypotension. Single-artery infarct, usually middle cerebral artery (MCA) or frontal, occurs without any obvious disease or risk factors. Newborns appear normal at birth, but repetitive focal or generalised seizures occur at any time during the first 4–7 days of life. It may present as a weakness of one side, which is sometimes very difficult to diagnose, but repeat examination for babies who present with focal or generalised seizures will help to elicit early weaknesses. There is a risk that 20–40% of these children will develop either hemiplegia or subtle hemiplegia. The rest usually will be normal, but all depends on the area involved and how severe the early presentation was.

Presentation with weakness and seizure is usually not a good sign. Cranial CT with contrast or MRI is very important to demonstrate the area of infarction and to see if it is associated with any parenchymal bleed. US is also very helpful in the case of a large MCA infarct. The follow-up may show ventricular dilation or porencephaly contralateral to the hemiparesis. Maternal use of cocaine during pregnancy can cause infarction. Anticonvulsants are effective in controlling seizures. Phenobarbitone is more effective in the early days, with a later switch to other anti-epileptic drugs (AED) in patients with intractable seizures. Only 20–40% of these patients may need long-term anticonvulsant treatment, and surgery for patients with epilepsy and intractable seizures should be considered.

Case 21

A 10-year-old child presented with a history of bruising, which spread over his legs and arms. He is an only child with no family history of illness. He was on a school trip to the south of Italy 2 weeks ago, when he felt sick for 1 day. His mother had four miscarriages, two of them due to chromosomal abnormalities. He has complained of leg pains in the past and recently he was diagnosed as having migraine, which responded to simple analgesia. He is afebrile and there is no organomegaly. His urine shows RBCs and no pus cells. The test results are:

Hb	12.5 g/dl
WCCs	$8.4 \times 10^9/l$
PLT	$15 \times 10^9/l$
PTT	38 s (control 35–50 s)
BT	1 min (control 30–60 s)
Film	PLT small in size

1. What is the most likely diagnosis?
2. What are three possible causes?
3. What is the treatment?

Case 22

A girl presented who is described by her mother as 'unsteady on her feet' and has had poor weight gain since the age of 3 years. Her early development was within the normal range and there were no previous concerns. She is now 6 years old, is still having a problem with her gait and is not able to ride a bicycle. Sometimes her older brother has described her as a 'drunken child'. She was admitted to hospital 1 year ago with bad chest infection, and was treated with i.v. antibiotics and had fluid drained from her lungs. Both parents are healthy, although her father had a problem with his eyes that required surgery. Her younger sister is healthy. The family lives in an old house with damp and a falling ceiling. She used to be bright and active, but now is withdrawn and sleepy, and not as noisy as before. She swings when she walks and has marked tremor in her hands. Her eyes started to turn red in last 3 months and treatment for conjunctivitis was prescribed by her GP. No other abnormalities were found on systemic and general examination. The test results are:

ESR	90 mm/hour
Hb	7.2 g/dl
Hb electrophoresis	No haemoglobinopathy
Ret	1.2%
Ca	1.78 mmol/l
Inorganic phosphate	1.97 mmol/l
Vitamin D	10 mmol/l

1. What is the most likely diagnosis?
2. Which four other blood tests will help the diagnosis?
3. What other clinical manifestations may develop?

Case 23

A family of Middle Eastern origin presented with their 3-year-old son, who has become more pale and tired in the last 7 days. He suffered a URTI 1 week ago and has since never regained his original colour. His parents are first cousins and have an older child, a girl, who is well. The patient had always been described as a boy with 'waxy skin' as he is pale. His eye movement is chaotic and his mother describes him as a 'clumsy child' and has said that in the last 2 weeks he has fallen a lot. He has not participated in any games with his sister or anyone, as he gets tired very easily. He is on the 3rd centile for weight and 10th centile for height. His cousin died from a brain tumour 3 years ago at the age of 3 years. His parents visit their homeland twice every year and his grandmother suffers from chronic arthritis.

He looks pale, with a distended abdomen and liver measuring 2 cm, with a possible renal mass. The fundi are normal and there is no joint problem. He is anaemic with normal platelet and white cell counts. His liver function and renal function are normal. The alpha-fetoprotein level is within the normal range.

1. Which three investigations can be performed to help the diagnosis, and in what order?
   a   Blood film
   b   Abdominal US
   c   I.v. pyelography (IVP)
   d   Abdominal and chest CT
   e   Bone marrow biopsy
   f   Abdominal mass biopsy
   g   Hepatitis B serology
   h   Hepatitis C serology
   i   Chromosomal study
   j   Urinary vanillylmandelic and homovanillic acid
2. What is the diagnosis?
3. List three steps of management
   a   Hyperhydration
   b   Adrenocorticotrophic hormone (ACTH)
   c   Oral allopurinol
   d   I.v. antibiotics
   e   Oral hydrocortisone
   f   Remove abdominal mass
   g   Insert urinary catheter
   h   Nil per mouth
   i   I.v. antifungal agent
   j   Blood transfusion
   k   Transfer to specialised oncology unit
   l   Peritoneal dialysis

Case 24

A 7-year-old boy with a history of recurrent bruising presented to his family doctor. His mother also suffers from recurrent bruises. He was born at term with no neonatal problems. He had nasal bleeds at the ages of 5 and 6 years. He cannot play football, as he gets tired and will suffer from bad bruises. His two older brothers are well and healthy, as is his father. There are two bruises on his thigh following his attempt to climb a tree. No other abnormalities are found on systemic or general examination. His mother had a termination of pregnancy for reason of fetal cardiac abnormalities. The family owns a horse and the boy looks after it. The boy was referred to hospital 3 months ago for a 1 × 1 cm cervical lymphadenopathy, which is still there. The bruises are becoming more frequent and he feels upset not to be allowed to go swimming with his friend or play football, as these cause more bruises. His WCC, haemoglobin level and lymph node biopsy were reported as normal. There is no rash and a normal MSU. All joints are intact and are not painful.

1. What other tests should be carried out?
   a Blood film
   b Bone marrow aspiration
   c Chromosomal study
   d Bleeding time
   e PTT
   f INR
   g Platelet count
   h Liver function test
   i PT
2. What is the diagnosis?
   a Haemophilia A
   b Glens syndrome
   c TAR syndrome
   d ALL
   e von Willebrand disease
   f Henoch–Schönlein purpura
   g Ehlers–Danlos syndrome
   h Christmas disease
   i Aplastic anaemia
3. What two other blood tests should you carry out?
   a Factor VIII assay
   b Factor X assay
   c Bone marrow
   d Chromosomal study
   e Platelets ristocetin aggregation test
   f von Willebrand factors assay
   g Bleeding time
   h Fibrinogen level

Case 25

The following are the blood results from a 3-year-old child with diarrhoea and vomiting that has continued for the last 12 hours. His mother suggested that his stool looks mucousy, with streaks of a reddish mixture. He has stopped drinking and eating, and is not happy. His HR is 110 b.p.m., RR 40/min and BP 110/60 mmHg. He looks pale and shut down but his capillary refill is < 2 s centrally. His mother had a similar illness 2 weeks ago but recovered within 3 days. His doctor prescribed Dioralyte and analgesia. His urine output is minimal. He was admitted to his local hospital for further management. The test results are:

Blood

Na	125 mmol/l
K	5.3 mmol/l
Cl	90 mmol/l
Urea	21 mmol/l
Cr	230 mmol/l
HCO_3	14

Urine

Na	10
Osmolality	700 mosmol/l
Blood culture	Negative
MSU	Negative
Abdominal US	No abnormalities

1. What other investigations should be carried out to help in diagnosis and management?
    a   Hb
    b   INR
    c   PTT
    d   PT
    e   Blood film
    f   Platelet count
    g   LFT
    h NH_4
    i   Abdominal CT
    j   IVP
    k   Blood gas
2. What is the diagnosis, judging from the blood test?
3. Which four steps should form the initial management of this child, and in what order?
    a   Fluid restriction to 300 ml/m² of surface area
    b   I.v. antibiotics
    c   Urinary output to be added to total fluid
    d   4-hourly U&E
    e   Transfer to specialised unit
    f   Platelet transfusion
    g   Blood transfusion
    h   Peritoneal dialysis

i   Plasmapheresis
j   I.v. vitamin K
k   Correct acidosis

Case 26

An 8-year-old girl presented with a history of back pain for the last 7 days and an inability to walk in the last 4 hours (she was all right and walked to school that morning). She had a mild fever and was feeling sick, and there have been no other symptoms in the last 24 hours. She was on a coach trip to France with her school 2 weeks ago and developed a very bad cold on the second day. She recovered within 2 days and was able to do most of the visiting with the school to various places, including the Eiffel tower in Paris. There are no other concerns. Now she says she 'can't feel her legs', even when her mother presses hard on them. The reflexes in her lower limbs are brisk and the plantar upgoing. She is not responding to pain or touch in her lower limbs up to the suprapubic region. All cranial nerves are intact and examination of the upper limbs and other systems is normal. Her bladder is palpable, as she has not passed any urine in the last 18 hours. The test results are (cerebrospinal fluid [CSF]):

WCC	50 (all lymphocytes)
Protein	1.2 g/l
Glucose	2.8 mmol/l (serum 5.6 mmol/l)
Gram stain	No organism
C/S	Negative
PCR, HSV/polio/TB/*Mycoplasma*/ Enterovirus	All negative
IgG oligoclonal antibodies	Not found
Spinal X-ray	Normal

1.   What is the most likely diagnosis?
   a   Spinal cord compression
   b   Syringomyelia
   c   Acute transverse myelitis
   d   MS
   e   Guillain–Barré syndrome
   f   Occlusive vascular disease
   g   UTI
   h   Spinal shock syndrome
2.   What are the other most useful investigations?
   a   Spinal CT
   b   Spinal MRI
   c   Spinal and cranial MRI
   d   Cranial MRI
   e   Peripheral nerve conduction study
   f   DNA double strand
   g   Cerebral angiography
   h   Bone marrow biopsy

    i   EMG
    j   Urinary VMA
3.   What is the immediate treatment?
    a   High-dose pulses of methylprednisolone until recovery,
         followed by oral corticosteroids for 6 weeks
    b   High dose of oral prednisolone for 6 weeks
    c   IVIG
    d   Plasmapheresis
    e   Surgical cord decompression
    f   Intensive physiotherapy
    g   Bladder catheterisation care

Case 27

A 7-year-old girl presented with a history of increasing axillary
hair as well as pubic hair. Her mother's period started at the age
of 13 years. In the last few days she started to have early morning
sickness with abdominal pain. Her weight is on the 50th centile and
her height on the 75th centile; her mother's height is on the 90th
centile. Her pubic hair is stage T3, axillary, stage 2 and breasts,
stage 1. She has never had any vaginal bleeding. She lives with her
mother and spends 2 weekends per month with her father, who is
married and has two children with his new partner. Sometimes she
wakes up at night, complaining of abdominal pain and comes to her
mother, telling her about her nightmares. She attends swimming
youth club and finds it difficult to change her clothes in the
changing room. Her GP assured her mother that it is nothing to
worry about when he saw her for the first time 6 months ago about
the pubic hair. Most of the time a childminder will pick her up from
school, as her mother works as a full-time journalist. The test results
are:

Testosterone	1.0 nmol/l	(1–2 nmol/l)
Cortisol	220 nmol/l	(140–7000 nmol/l)
TSH	2.7 mU/l	(0.35–5.00 mU/l)
Free thyroxine	14 pmol/l	(9.0–19.0 pmol/l)
FSH	21.2 u/l (follicular phase)	(4–15 u/l)
LH	29 u/l (follicular phase)	(4–15 u/l)
Oestradiol	450 pmol/l	(< 350 pmol/l)

1.   Which three other investigations would help the diagnosis?
    a   LH/FSH stimulation test
    b   Chromosomal study
    c   Abdominal US
    d   Histosalpingography
    e   Abdominal CT
    f   Urinary 17-hydroxyprogesterone
    g   Glucagon-suppression test
    h   Cranial MRI
    i   Short Synacthen test
2.   What are the three differential diagnoses?

Case 28

The following CSF results are from a 3-year-old boy who presented to A&E with a mild temperature and generalised tonic–clonic seizures. His mother is a nurse and started him on amoxycillin 4 days ago for tonsillitis. He kept on having a mild temperature; his appetite improved but he was still lethargic and kept crying from time to time without a reason. His seizure stopped after 5 min but he was still drowsy. His temperature in Casualty was 36.4°C, his HR 150 b.p.m., RR 22/min, and Sat 99% on 5 l/min oxygen via a facemask. His mother said he suffers from tonsillitis quite often, up to 3 times each year, and had one bout of left upper lobe pneumonia in the past at age 6 months. He started having generalised tonic–clonic seizures, and 5 mg rectal diazepam was given and a cranial CT was carried out. He maintained his airway and was transferred to the ward after he was started on antibiotics and acyclovir. His CSF test results are:

WCCs	120 (60% lymphocytes)
Protein	200 g/l
Glucose	1.1 mmol/l
Serum glucose	5.1 mmol/l
Gram stain	Negative
RBCs	0

1.   What abnormalities are visible on his cranial CT?

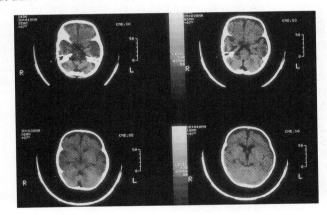

  a   Cerebral oedema
  b   Middle cerebral artery infarct
  c   Subarachnoid haemorrhage
  d   Increase in subdural space
  e   No abnormalities on both scans
  f   Basal ganglia infarction
  g   Absent corpus callosum

2. What other single test should you carry out?
    a   Mantoux test
    b   Igs (immunoglobulins)
    c   Lymphocyte subset
    d   HIV test
    e   Herpes simplex PCR on CSF
    f   CSF PCR for *Staphylococcus*, *Streptococcus* and *Neisseria*
    g   EEG
    h   MRI scan
3. What is the diagnosis?

Case 29

A 5-month-old baby presented with a history of recurrent chest infections for the last 4 weeks. He has not gained weight for the last 4 weeks (his weight is on the 3rd centile and his birthweight was on the 25th centile). There is no diarrhoea or vomiting. He had three CXRs and was reported to have hyperinflated lungs. He has just started solids, which he likes. He looks puffy, pale and thin. He is hypotonic and has stopped smiling. His abdomen is soft and a mild wheeze was discovered during a chest examination. There is no family history of chest or gut problems and his parents are not related. This is their first baby and there were no neonatal problems. He has fed very well from the first day of life and passed meconium in the first 18 hours after birth. He is anaemic and a sweat test showed Na of 46 mmol/l (N = 20–60 mmol/l) of reasonable sweat. There are no other concerns and both parents are healthy. There is no family history of any illnesses. The Igs, stool for reducing substances, platelet count and urine culture were all reported as normal.

1. What are the four differential diagnoses, and in what order would you list them?
    a   Lactose intolerance
    b   Gastro-esophageal reflux (GOR)
    c   Tracheo-oesophageal fistulae
    d   Cystic fibrosis
    e   Schwachman syndrome
    f   Protein cows' milk intolerance
    g   Autoimmune deficiency syndrome
    h   Congenital cystic lung disease
    i   Congenital enteropathy
2. Which other three tests should be carried out?
    a   Sweat test with hydrofludrocortisone suppression
    b   Hydrogen breath test
    c   IgG subclasses
    d   Bronchoscopy and lavage
    e   HIV test
    f   pH study
    g   Chest CT
    h   Barium swallow

i   Skin allergy test
j   Upper and lower GIT endoscopy
k   DNA linkage study for CF
l   Faecal elastasis

Case 30

A 14-year-old boy had blood taken by his GP for investigation of enlarged cervical lymph glands. He started having generalised tonic–clonic seizures 2 min later. This lasted for 2 min, followed by headache. There is no family history of epilepsy and he had a similar episode when he attended a dental appointment for a tooth extraction. Blood was taken, including serum glucose, Ca, Mg and electrolytes, and there were no abnormalities found. He has a hyperpigmented birthmark measuring 7 × 5 cm on his left scapula. He is also wearing glasses for a lazy left eye and is under follow-up by an ophthalmologist. He had an EEG as well as an MRI scan, carried out privately. The brain MRI and asleep and awake EEGs were normal.

1. What is the most likely diagnosis?
    a   Reflex anoxic seizures
    b   Vasovagal attack
    c   Panic attack
    d   Idiopathic generalised seizure
    e   Hyperkeplexia
    f   Idiopathic focal epilepsy
    g   Tics

ANSWERS 21–30

Case 21

1. Idiopathic thrombocytopenia purpura (ITP)
2. Idiopathic
    Viral infection
    Autoimmune/drugs
3. Supportive with regular follow-up

Thrombocytopenia in children

This is an autoimmune disease that affects children at any age. Neonatal thrombocytopenia is associated with intrauterine growth retardation (IUGR); congenital infection; maternal SLE; maternal ITP; maternal haemolysis, elevated liver enzymes and low platelets (HELLP) syndrome; sepsis; Fanconi pancytopenia; TAR (thrombocytopenia and absence radius) syndrome; Wiskott–Aldrich syndrome; neonatal leukaemia; and neuroblastoma. In children it is usually idiopathic, but exclusion of malignancy, infection, connective-tissue disorders (e.g. SLE), viral illnesses (e.g. adenovirus, B_{12}/folate deficiency, haemolytic uraemic syndrome, Kasbach–Merritt syndrome, endocarditis and aplastic anaemia) is important. The ITP-affected child usually presents with bruises 2–4 weeks after viral illness. The disorder is characterised by an increased amount of IgG on the platelets. The reticuloendothelial cells within the spleen will usually clear the IgG-coated platelets. Easy bruising, purpura and petechial rashes are the acute presenting features. Epistaxis is the presenting feature in some patients. Others present with mucous membrane bleeding (very small numbers). Some patients may have splenomegaly but in the majority general and systemic examinations will be normal. The blood film will show small platelets, and bone marrow aspiration is not indicated unless suspicion of malignancy is raised. Recovery of platelet count within 1 month occurs in most patients and 75% of patients will recover within 6 months. If there is no mucous membrane bleeding or risk of ICB (intracranial bleeding), there is no need to treat the patient with IVIG. Platelet transfusion is not indicated unless there is active bleeding and the platelet count is very low. General advice about avoiding accidents and contact sports for the period of low platelet count is very important. This disease will persist for more than 5 years in fewer than 5% of affected individuals and splenectomy is not indicated in the majority of these cases. The mortality rate is very low in patients with ITP.

Case 22

1.   Ataxia telangiectasia
2.   Ig
       Cellular DNA
       Chromosomes
       Cranial MRI
3.   Malignancies (lymphomas)
       Bone marrow failure

Ataxia telangiectasia

This is a multisystem disorder affecting the central nervous system (CNS) and immune system. It can be transmitted through autosomal recessive inheritance. The genetic marker has been located on the long arm of chromosome 11. The manifestation can begin as early as the first year of life, with ataxia. The child usually presents with clumsiness and frequent falls, which become progressive. Sometimes this may be accompanied by chorioathetotic movement. Oculomotor apraxia is present in 90% of patients and can be early. Intellectual development will be normal in early life but will decline slowly as the child grows up. Telangiectasia usually develops in years 2–4 of life and sometimes at the age of 10. It appears as a bloodshot bulbar conjunctiva. It also appears on the upper part of the ears, on the flexor surface of limbs, and as a butterfly distribution on the face. Frequent lung infection can be very serious, and indicaties problems with the immune system in these patients. There are disturbances in both B- and T-helper cells. Serum and saliva IgE is absent in 70–80% of patients. IgE is absent in 90% but the IgM level is elevated. The thymus is less well developed and the alpha-fetoprotein level is high in the majority of patients. There is an increased incidence of malignancy, in particular lymphoma and lymphoblastic leukaemia; at least two-thirds of these patients die before the age of 20 years. The diagnosis is usually made on the basis of clinical situation and signs. Genetic study as well as increased DNA breakdown when exposed to radiation are other useful tests that can be carried out. Regular follow-up and family support are very important. Genetic counselling are vital and prenatal diagnosis can be done.

Case 23

1. j   Urinary vanillylmandelic acid
   d   Abdominal and chest CT
   f   Abdominal mass biopsy
2. Myoclonic encephalopathy (neuroblastoma syndrome)
3. e   Oral hydrocortisone
   c   Oral allopurinol
   k   Transfer to specialised oncology unit

Myoclonic encephalopathy (neuroblastoma syndrome)

This is characterised by chaotic eye movements (dancing eye syndrome), myoclonic ataxia and encephalopathy. It may occur idiopathically or secondary to occult neuroblastoma. The outcome is usually the same, whatever the mode of presentation. It can present at any time from 6 months to 6 years of age. Clumsiness or abnormal eye movement is usually the first presentation, which may take a week or longer before being brought to the attention of a medical professional. More than half will present with irritability and behavioural changes that indicate encephalopathy. There is a spontaneous, conjugated, irregular jerking of the eyes in all directions, which is called opsoclonus. This eye movement persists during sleep and is more severe when the child is agitated or tired. The diagnosis can be made based on clinical background, and looking for the cause is important. Looking for urinary homovanillic acid and vanillylmandelic acid is very important, as is MIBG scan on bone marrow to stage the neuroblastoma. A CT or MRI of the chest and abdomen, looking for the occult neuroblastoma, can be carried out. Either ACTH or oral corticosteroids provide partial or complete relief of symptoms in 80% of patients, including those with neuroblastoma. Partial or complete remission of the neurological syndrome may occur regardless of whether neuroblastoma is present. If a neuroblastoma is present, it should be removed.

Case 24

1. a, b, d–i, All except a chromosomal study
2. von Willebrand disease
3. a   Factor VIII restocetin assay
      von Willebrand factors assay

von Willebrand disease

This usually presents as mucocutaneous bleeding, but other features may arise. Bruising after trauma is another mode of presentation. It is inherited as an autosomal dominant disorder but homozygous cases do occur. There is failure in factor VIIIc, VIII RAG, and VIII VWF, and fibrinogen synthesis. The bleeding time and PTT are prolonged, and fibrinogen, PT and TT are normal. Ristocetin-induced platelet aggregation is impaired because factor VIII VWF potentiates platelet adherence to the subendothelial connective tissue. Epistaxis is a problem in patients with von Willebrand disease. Treatment with DDAVP is useful in raising VIII VWF in most types. Cryoprecipitate, nasal cautery and tranexamic acid are helpful.

Case 25

1. e   Blood film
      d, c, b, PT, PTT, INR
      f   Platelet count
      i   Abdominal CT
      k   Blood gas
      a   Hb
2. Renal failure
3. a   Fluid restriction to 300 ml/m² of surface area
      c   Urinary output to be added to total fluid
      b   I.v. antibiotics
      e,   Transfer to specialised unit

Haemolytic uraemic syndrome

This is characterised by renal failure, thrombocytopenia and micro-angiopathic anaemia. It affects children at any age and there are two types. The endemic type, which affects infants and young children, usually follows diarrhoea. It has a good prognosis and many cases are missed, as presentation can be mild. The sporadic type can affect older children and no cause can be found. The prognosis is poor if it is not detected early and treated effectively. A blood film will show ghost cells and red cells that look as if some parts are missing or have been 'bitten off' by something. The platelet number is low; the bleeding time will be long but the PT and PTT are normal, as is the level of fibrinogen. Fresh plasma may help to restore lost volume, and plasmapheresis, aspirin, and heparin are useful but not very effective. The treatment that will save renal function is dialysis, and can be peritoneal or haemodialysis. Peritoneal dialysis is much easier to perform and no machine or highly skilled training is required. There is no risk of transmitted diseases, but it may increase the risk of peritonitis, viscus penetration, pleural effusion and sepsis. The indication for dialysis in renal failure includes uraemic CNS signs such as irritability, seizures or semi-coma, biochemical disturbances (hyperkalaemia, hyponatraemia, metabolic acidosis, and hypercalcaemia). A urea level of > 60 mmol/l is another indication for dialysis.

Case 26

1. c   Acute transverse myelitis
2. c   Spinal and cranial MRI
   e   Peripheral nerve conduction study
3. a   High dose of methylprednisolone until recovery, followed by oral corticosteroids for 6 weeks
   f   Intensive physiotherapy
   g   Bladder catheterisation care

Acute transverse myelitis

This is characterised by signs of lesions of both motor and sensory tracts on both sides of the spinal cord. Many disorders will cause this condition, e.g. postinfectious myelitis, multiple sclerosis, vascular insufficiency, direct viral infection, X-irradiation and vascular malformation. There is inflammation and demyelination on perivenous distribution. The most common cause remains unknown, and it often follows viral infection (with CMV, HSV, hepatitis A and adenovirus). Lyme disease, *Mycoplasma* pneumonia and typhoid vaccine can also cause transverse myelitis. Most cases occur in children older than 5 years, but it may occur at any age. The first symptoms to occur are pain in the back, followed by paraplegia with sphincter paralysis, and marked sensory disturbances. Sometimes it may evolve over days with a history of paraesthesia, then followed by weakness and urinary retention. Some patients may have meningeal irritation with neck stiffness. It is characterised by flaccid paralysis with pyramidal tract involvement. There are gross sensory disturbances with more pain, impaired sensation and loss of sense of position. It is very difficult to localise the sensory disturbance level, but most motor and sensory disturbances occur in the thoracic regions (in 80% of cases). Respiratory involvement occurs in one-fifth of patients. The CSF will show pleocytosis and a high protein level in only 25% of patients. Spinal and cranial MRI scans are important to rule out compression lesions. Moderate swelling of the cord may be present and there are increased signals on T_2-weighted MRI. The majority (60%) of patients will make a good recovery. Less than 10% may develop MS and 10–20% will fail to improve. The more severe the state at presentation, the worse the prognosis. Treatment is usually supportive, and a high dose of methylprednisolone will help to reduce the swelling. Treating the cause is also helpful.

Case 27

1. c   Abdominal US
    f   Urinary 17-hydroxyprogesterone
    b   Chromosomal study
2. Premature adrenarch
    21-Hydroxylase deficiency
    Intersex

Ambiguous genitalia

This is one of the commonest congenital abnormalities where gender of a baby cannot be decided. It is very important when this problem is discovered that it is dealt with accurately and sensitively. It is important not to call the baby 'he' or 'she' and to ask the parents to call the baby 'baby Smith' and so on. The external genitalia develop from mesodermal thickening on either side of the urogenital sinus, the genital folds. In the absence of testosterone, or absence of response to testosterone, the genital folds fuse anteriorly to form the genital tubercle and then enlarge slightly to form the clitoris. Production of dihydrotestosterone from the Leydig cells of the testis results in enlargement of the genital tubercle and formation of the penis. The genital swelling in the female develops into the labia, while in the male it fuses in the midline to develop the urethra and scrotum.

Ambiguous genitalia may range from masculinization of a female fetus or less commonly inadequate masculinization of a male fetus to true hermaphroditism. The latter results in an enlarged clitoris/phallus, a urethral opening anywhere, abnormal genital swellings to form labia/scrotal sacs and occasionally a vaginal opening. If there is a positive test result on attempting to feel for the scrotum then masculinization of the fetus has occured. The principal cause of masculinization is congenital adrenal hyperplasia, and this should be considered as soon as possible because treatment can be given. Other causes may include maternal ingestion of androgens and maternal Cushing's disease. In the male, ambiguous genitalia are less common and may be due to true hermaphroditism, where testicular and ovarian tissues are found. In the undervirilised male with ambiguous genitalia, testicular tissue can be found. The diagnosis of both of these conditions can be made when the baby is examined under GA, lapratomy and gonadal biopsy. Congenital adrenal hyperplasia should be ruled out before carrying out these examinations.

Investigation of babies with congenital adrenal hyperplasia should include chromosomal (karyotyping) study, abdominal and pelvic US, 17-alpha-hydroxyprogesterone ($\uparrow$), testosterone ($\uparrow$), pregnanetriol ($\uparrow$), K ($\uparrow$) and reduced Na.

Genetic counselling and intersex clinics should be offered to the parents of these patients, and the decision to register the baby can be delayed until all tests are carried out.

Case 28

1. e   No abnormalities on cranial CT
2. b   Ig's
3.   Partially treated bacterial meningitis

Partially treated bacterial meningitis

Bacterial meningitis can present in different ways, but the commonest is with fever, irritability, a bulging fontanelle and infants that have stopped wanting to feed. In older children photophobia and meningeal signs can also be present, with a high temperature and headache. Oral antibiotics and poor compliance by parents may lead to partially treated meningitis. The symptoms will reoccur after stopping antibiotics or if an inadequate dosage is given. Irritability, a bulging fontanelle and fever will continue, as can headache with or without meningeal irritation. The CSF will show a high WCC with predominant lymphocytes, low glucose and high protein. No organism will be seen and cultures are usually negative. PCR for bacterial infection will be helpful. Treatment is by a 7-day course of i.v. antibiotics, with cephalosporins being the drugs of choice, although a combination of penicillin and gentamicin when cephalosporins are not available is a good combination. Sometimes it is very difficult to rule out tubercular meningitis, but the CSF protein will not be very high in partially treated meningitis. The clinical picture is different, with insidious progress of symptoms for tubercular meningitis over several weeks. If in doubt, it is important to test for tubercular meningitis.

Case 29

1. d   Cystic fibrosis
        Pancolitis
   a   Lactose intolerance
   b   GOR
2. a   Sweat test with hydrofludrocortisone suppression
   k   DNA linkage study for CF
   l   Faecal elastasis

Sweat test

This is one of the diagnostic tests for CF. It can be carried out safely at any age but in premature babies it will be very difficult. It is important to collect the right amount of sweat, and any equivocal results should be repeated with corticosteroid suppression as well as doing a genetic study and faecal elastasis. If the clinical suspicion of CF is very high and all tests are still equivocal, then axiliary voltage study should be done at a specialist centre.

Indications for a sweat test include a family history of CF, patients who failed to thrive, and those with both GIT and respiratory symptoms. Meconium ileus in the neonatal period and a distant relative who is a known case should raise clinical suspicion. A 100 mg quantity of sweat is no longer required in places where the macroduct system is used as opposed to the older methods, in which evaporation led to falsely elevated sweat electrolyte levels. Sweat testing can be performed in babies who are > 48 hours old. There is a normal range of sweat sodium of < 40 mmol/l; the test will need to be repeated if the sweat Na result is between 40 and 60 mmol/l, and if > 60 mmol/l, the diagnosis is CF. The diagnosis of CF should be based on the result of two sweat tests, not one. A false-positive sweat test can be associated with dermatitis/eczema, coeliac disease, untreated hypothyroidism, malnutrition, and flucloxacillin use. A CF diagnosis should always be made on the basis of high clinical suspicion.

Case 30

1. a   Reflex anoxic seizures

Anoxic seizures

These are due to cortical hypoxic failure of energy metabolism as a result of anoxia and hypoxia. They may follow bradycardia < 40 b.p.m., tachycardia > 150 b.p.m., asystole > 60 s, or systolic BP < 50 mmHg. Cortical hypoxia results in loss of consciousness and postural hypotonia. Anoxic seizures can be due to several mechanisms, which include breathholding, obstructive apnoea, Valsalva manoeuvre, cardiac diseases, fainting attacks and brain compression. Reflex anoxic seizures result from emotional stimuli, or stress, minor pain or injury. This is actually a syncope attack followed by seizure. It is usually described as the patient going pale, with eyes that may be deviated, and the pulse slow. In some cases true epileptic attacks occur, induced by hypoxia. Many of these attacks have an abrupt onset and tonic clonic movement and the patient becomes rigid. Postictal confusion is common and can be familial, as in vasovagal syncope. Reassurance is usually what should be offered, as well as investigation if the history suggests that this is necessary.

Case 31

A 10-year-old boy presented with a history of lethargy and abnormal behaviour at school. He is taking iron tablets for iron-deficiency anaemia, which was diagnosed by his doctor. The boy is the only child in the family; they live in a three-bedroomed Victorian house. He is withdrawn and does not want to talk. He has been described as a 'violent child' by his mother on several occasions in the last 3 months, and has been expelled from a school club because of his behaviour. Sometimes he complains of headache, with fuzzy vision. His eyes were checked twice and no abnormalities could be found by his local optometrist. A fundi examination during this admission showed papilloedema. Twice a year, he visits his father who has lived in another country for the last 4 years. His best friend left him, as they had arguments all the time in the last 3 months over simple things. The boy's mother has had to give up her work until his problem is sorted out. He threatened her that one day he would jump from the first floor window, where he sits most of the time. He stopped taking his iron tablets and has also started losing weight. He wakes up at night shouting and complaining of headache, which has been resolved by analgesia on several occasions. The boy looks withdrawn and makes no eye contact. He hates school and does not want to go back. He wants to go and live with his father.

All aspects of the systemic examination are normal. All cranial nerves are intact but he does not like to have a light shone into his eyes. A fundi examination shows papilloedema and no other abnormalities. His BP is 120/75 mmHg, HR 70 b.p.m., and RR 20/min. Other test results are:

Hb	8.7 g/dl
MCV	45 fl
MCHC	25 g/dl
PLT	357×10^9/l
BS	4.5 mmol/l
Urine	Proteinuria and phosphaturia

1. Is his abdominal X-ray (shown on the next page) abnormal and if so, what are the abnormalities?
   a   Normal
   b   Shows evidence of constipation
   c   Abnormal

After admission, he had a cranial MRI, which was reported as normal. After midnight, he started to have generalised tonic–clonic seizures for 5 min, which stopped after administration of rectal diazepam. There were no more seizures and an EEG was carried out urgently, which also was reported to show no epileptiform activity. His behaviour fluctuated and a decision was made to treat him as having encephalitis. All his films were reviewed by a radiologist, who said he may have ureteral stones and a calcified lesion in the bladder.

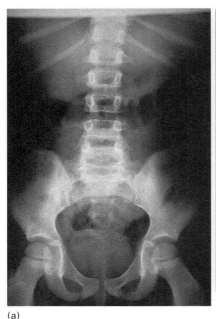

(a)

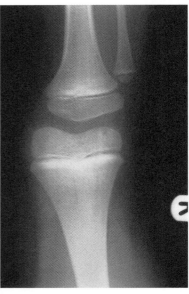

(b)

2. What single test should be carried out?
    a Abdominal US
    b IVP
    c Cystoscopy
    d Ferritin level
    e Lead level
    f VMA
    g Barium swallow
    h Urine toxicology
    i LP
    j Ammonia level
    k Mantoux test
3. Which other two investigations should be carried out?
    a Blood film
    b Urinary copper level
    c Long-bone X-ray
    d Abdominal CT
    e CSF for HSV PCR
    f Repeat EEG
4. What is the diagnosis?

He was treated and 6 weeks later another blood test was taken, which showed that he still had the same problem, even though there had been some improvement in his behaviour and he had attended school in the preceding 2 weeks.

5. What should the management plan be?
   a   Admit to hospital until he finishes the course of treatment
   b   Contact the Environmental Health Officer
   c   Refer to psychiatrist
   d   Inform social services and child protection team
   e   Start treatment again with strict supervision by a community care team

Case 32

A 6-month-old infant girl presented with a history of jaundice and poor feeding for the last 15 days. The liver measurement is 3 cm and the spleen is tipped. Both parents are refugees from Kosovo, and there is no consanguinity. An older sibling, aged 3 years, is healthy, and there is no family history of such an illness. The father is suffering from recurrent renal calculi. No metabolic cause could be found for his problem. The girl is also hypotonic, with a large, protuberant abdomen. She is passing normal stool and her weight is on the 10th centile.

Hb	10.3 g/dl
WCC	$16 \times 10^9/l$
PLT	$90 \times 10^9/l$
Alk. Alk. PhPh	200 mmol/l
γGT	300 mmol/l
ALT	180 IU/l
Alb	20 IU/l
Total protein	60 g/l
Bilirubin	200 μmol/l
Conjugated bilirubin	80 μmol/l
PTT	140 s
PT	90 s
Urine	Glucosuria, protein ++, and aminoaciduria
Stool	Normal in colour
Alpha-fetoprotein	High

1. Which four investigations should be carried out and in which order?
   a   Blood gas
   b   Hepatitis B serology
   c   Hepatitis C serology
   d   EBV serology
   e   Human immune deficiency virus (HIV) antibodies
   f   Abdominal US
   g   Bone marrow aspiration
   h   Blood film

     i   Liver biopsy
     j   Caeruloplasmin level
2.   Which two abnormalities appear on the wrist X-ray and photo?

All serology came back as negative and she was given FFP and vitamin K. She was referred to a metabolic team for further testing and they suggested some tests to be carried out locally.

3.   Which order of other investigations may help the diagnosis?
     a   Corrected calcium
     b   Phosphorus
     c   Vitamin D level
     d   Chromosomes
     e   AAs
     f   Liver biopsy
     g   White cell enzyme
     h   Bone marrow aspiration
     i   Urine for organic acids
     j   Parathyroid hormone level
4.   What is the diagnosis?

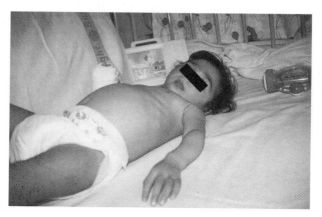

(a)

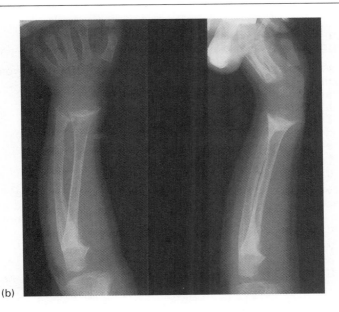

(b)

Case 33

An 11-year-old girl was referred to A&E with a history of haematuria. She lives with her father and two younger siblings. Her mother left home several years ago and the father cares for all of the children. The girl attends a mainstream school and her teacher is worried about her behaviour with other children, as she is not mixing with them and is using abusive language. She wants to run away from school and hates PE and swimming lessons. The male sports teacher manages the after-school club and thinks she would be a good swimmer. Her father does a part-time job at a local chip shop and never works at night. The girl was seen by a psychiatrist on a few occasions after concern was expressed about her running away from home, which is now settling. Her younger brother has a learning problem and attends the same school. An examination by her GP showed no evidence of organomegaly, anal fissure or valvovaginitis.

A urine dipstick is clear and a culture is negative. She was admitted to hospital 2 weeks ago with abdominal pain, which resolved and she was sent home with no arrangement for a follow-up. Social services were informed and a letter was sent to her GP.

PTT	34 s
TT1	1s
BT	35 s
INR	1.5
Hb	13 g/dl

PLT   180 × 10⁹/l
MCV   86 fl
MCHC   29 g/dl

1. What are the likely diagnoses and in what order would you select them?
    a   UTI
    b   Valvovaginitis
    c   Grumbling appendix
    d   Threadworms
    e   Ureterocoele
    f   Constipation
    g   CSA

She was admitted 2 weeks later, having taken an overdose of paracetamol in an attempt to kill herself. That day she was at a school club. She was treated for a drug overdose and her LFT was normal when tested on several occasions.

2. What should be the three steps of management?
    a   Admit her to a psychiatry unit
    b   Refer her to Social Services
    c   Carry out a forensic medical examination (FME)
    d   Refer her to a psychiatrist
    e   Temporary foster care
    f   Discharge her home
    g   Refer her to a child protection team

Case 34

A 4-day-old baby boy presented with cyanosis and shock. The Sat level was 70% in 10 l/min oxygen via a facemask. He was born vaginally at term and there were no problems in the first 3 days. Now he is not interested in his food and in the last 12 hours has begun to breathe heavily. There is no history of apnoea and he vomited once this morning. He sleeps in his cot by his parents' bed and the temperature outside is below 0°C. His antenatal scan shows no abnormalities and two other siblings are healthy. His RR is around 15/min and his HR is 100 b.p.m. His temperature, taken centrally, is 34°C; his BP is unrecordable, with a capillary refill time (CRT) of 4 s. He is mottled, cold and sleepy. His twin sister is very well and healthy. The baby's mother is a policewoman and his father is self-employed, and was still at work when the baby was brought to hospital. An i.v. cannula was inserted and blood was sent for analysis. The blood glucose level was 1.2 mmol/l, which was confirmed by laboratory results.

Blood glucose   1.2 mmol/l
CRP   59
U&E's   Normal
LFT's   Normal
Blood count showed neutrophilia

Arterial gas

pH	7.22
PCO_2	5.1 kpa
PO_2	4.5 kpa
$BCHO_3$	14
Be	−17

1. Which four urgent steps should be carried out?
   a   Immediate intubation and ventilation
   b   10 ml/kg of 0.9% NaCl given intravenously
   c   CXR
   d   Start i.v. antibiotics (benzylpenicillin and gentamicin)
   e   Full septic screen, including LP
   f   Naso-pharyngeal aspirate (NPA)
   g   Give prophylactic antibiotics to siblings and parents
   h   Echocardiography
2. What abnormalities are visible on the chest X-ray?

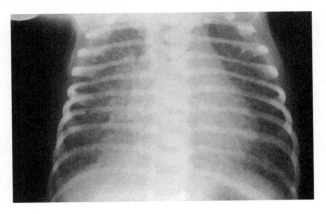

   a   Consolidation of left upper lobe
   b   Consolidation of right upper lobe
   c   Hyperinflation
   d   Bronchial wall thickening
   e   Collapse of right upper lobe
   f   No abnormalities

The baby was transferred to the PICU; his other blood tests came back and show:

TSH	150 mU/l
T4	12 mU/l
MSU	> 100 WCC
Nitrite	Negative

All blood, urine, and CSF tests are normal, as well as virology testing for herpes, adenovirus, and RSV.

Plasma and urinary AAs and urinary organic acids are normal, and the baby was taken off the ventilator, but still is not well. He was diagnosed as having sepsis and treated for 7 days with i.v. antibiotics.

3. What are two other possible causes?
    a Sepsis
    b Hypothyroidism
    c Chest infection
    d Metabolic disorder
    e Hypothermia
    f Complex heart lesions
    g Immune deficiency disorders
    h Encephalitis
    i Meningitis
    j CF
    k NAI

Case 35

A girl aged 12 years presented to A&E with a history of frequent headaches. The headaches usually occur during the daytime and sometimes in the early morning. There is no history of vomiting, falls, or abnormal movements. She is living with her grandmother and has been in the UK for only 9 months. Both parents live in Somalia. There is no previous history of illness. She is not taking any medication and her grandmother is healthy. There is no history of a high temperature or weight loss. Her headaches occasionally improve with paracetamol. The examination reveals no abnormalities, including fundi. Various blood tests were carried out and the results are:

Hb	13.4 g/dl
WWC	6.8 × 10⁹/l (N 42%, L 46%)
PLT	555 × 10⁹/l
CRP	< 5
ESR	21 mm/hour
LFT and U&Es	Within normal range

She was admitted for observation as she has been feeling sick since the morning. I.v. fluids were started, she slept all night and only required analgesia by lunchtime the next morning. She is still not drinking, the i.v. fluids have been stopped and she planned to go home by the early evening. Her headache got worse overnight and she did not sleep through the night, even after having been given three types of analgesia. The next morning, she is very weak and can't open her eyes or lift herself up. Her fundi are normal apart from a blurred half of the disc margin on the left. Her BP is 110/60 mmHg, HR 80 b.p.m., and RR 20/min.

1. Which three other investigations should be carried out and in what order?
    a CXR
    b Cranial CT

c   Viral serology
d   EEG
e   ECG
f   Urine toxicology
g   Abdominal US
h   Urinary VMA

2.   What abnormality appears on her cranial CT scan?

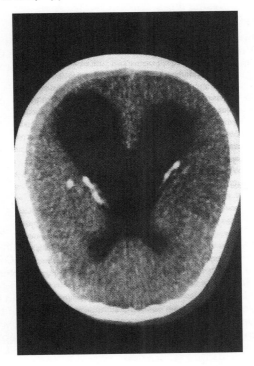

a   Dilated lateral ventricles
b   Dilated third ventricle
c   Dilated fourth ventricle
d   Lateral ventricular mass
e   Posterior fossa mass
f   Brainstem tumour
g   Cerebral oedema
h   Parieto-temporal attenuation
i   Internal capsule infarct
j   Hypothalamic infarct
k   Pontine infarct
l   Interventricular shunt in situ

3.   Which three procedures should be carried out to confirm the diagnosis and in what order would you place them?

   a   CSF for culture and sensitivity as well as PCR for *Mycobacterium*
   b   Refer to psychologist
   c   Cranial MRI
   d   EEG
   e   Mantoux test
   f   CXR
   g   *Mycoplasma* titres
   h   Transfer to neurosurgical ward for IVP shunt

Her CSF shows a protein level of 1.8 g/l, lymphocytosis, a glucose level of 2.1 mmol/l and a serum level of 6.7 mmol/l. A Gram stain was negative. Her MRI shows only dilated ventricles with meningeal irritation.

4.   What is the most likely diagnosis?
   a   Optic neuritis
   b   Guillain–Barré syndrome
   c   Brain tumour
   d   Tubercular meningitis
   e   Encephalomyelitis
   f   Brain abscess
   g   Autoimmune deficiency syndrome

Case 36

A pregnant woman was admitted to a labour ward at term with a history of vaginal bleeding and abdominal pain. The CTG for the baby showed late deceleration and an audible fetal heart sound of > 100 b.p.m. The fetal heart rate dropped 5 min later to 80 b.p.m. An emergency LSCS was done under general anaesthesia (GA). The fetal heart (FH) sound was audible but there is no record of the exact rate. The baby was delivered and remained unresponsive, with a HR of < 60 b.p.m. and no respiratory effort. The baby was floppy and dusky. Intubation was carried out and IPPV was given with 5 L/min oxygen. Within the first minute, the HR was back to > 100 b.p.m., a UVC was inserted and 10 ml/kg of 0.9% NaCl given. The baby was transferred to the NNU and put on a ventilator as there was no respiratory effort. The CMV test results are: P 20/4, IT 0.36, rate 50, FiO_2 100%, MAP 45, HR 135 b.p.m., and temperature 36.8°C. At the age of 60 min, the ventilation set-up was changed to rate 60 and pressure 24/4, and the FiO_2 remained at 100%. The test results are:

	pH	PCO_2(kPa)	PO_2(kPa)	HCO_3(kPa)	Be
Cord gas	6.889	12.4	4.0	9	−19
Age 30 min (V)	7.01	7.23	6.2	13	−11
Age 120 min (A)	7.24	6.01	7.3	15	−10
Age 3 hours (A)	7.36	7 .2	9.9	16	−2
Age 8 hours (A)	7.34	4.5	10.1	15	−2

1. What should be done at the age of 120 min?
   a   Reintubate
   b   CXR
   c   Half correction of acidosis by bicarbonate
   d   Cranial US
   e   Start nitrous oxide
   f   Start high-frequency oscillation (HFO)
   g   Increase RR to 70 and P to 26/5
   h   Give i.v. 10 ml/kg of 0.9% NaCl over 30 min

2. Why is the CO_2 level still high at age of 3 hours and all other gas normal parameters?
   a   Low RR
   b   Low IT
   c   Low PEEP
   d   Sepsis
   e   RDS
   f   From correction with bicarbonate
   g   Pneumothorax
   h   Blocked tube

The baby started having various types of seizures and was given a loading dose of phenobarbitone of 20 mg/kg.

3. What is this record called?

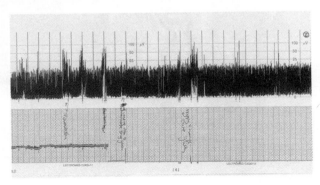

4. Is it normal or abnormal?

The baby was extubated at the age of 18 hours, a head US scan was taken, which shows generalised cerebral oedema, and 2 hours later he started having episodes of apnoea. Desaturated to 40% of PaO_2 and bradycardic to 60–70 b/min; he continued to fit. There were no changes in arterial gas and MAP, or oxygenation requirement.

5. What should your management plan be at this stage?
   a   Reintubate
   b   Reload with phenobarbitone
   c   Give maintenance treatment with phenobarbitone
   d   LP

e   Repeat septic screen
f   Repeat cranial US

The baby improved and there were no more episodes of apnoea. He started feeding the next morning and all medication stopped after 5 days; he was discharged home after 10 days.

6.   Which abnormalities appear on his MRI, taken 1 week later?

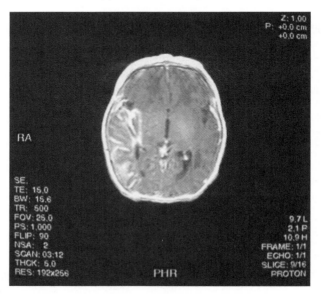

7.   What is the prognosis?
    a   Poor
    b   50% chance he will develop hemiplegia
    c   10–15% chance of normal development
    d   Good
    e   Speech problem

Case 37

A family doctor referred a 12-year-old girl with a history of illness for 7 days. She had mouth ulcers prior to her present febrile illness. She has had a high temperature on and off for the past 7 days. She developed cervical lymphadenopathy more on the left side as well as on her left axilla, and a small lymph node measuring 1 × 1 cm on the left of her groin. She also complained of a sore throat for the first 4 days and had puffy eyes, which have settled down now. She has never had conjunctivitis, or swollen palms or soles of her feet. Her spleen measures 1–2 cm below the left costal margin and she is very slim. On the seventh day, she developed a very small macular–papular rash, which is distributed on her back and upper chest. Her tonsils are large, inflamed, folliculated and covered with a white sheet, which is more on the right side than on the left.

Hb	13.1g/dl
WCC	7×10^9/l (50% N, 50% L)
PLT	250×10^9/l
Bilirubin	19 mmol/l (conjugated 1%)
ALT	32 IU/l
Alk. Ph	150 IU/l
CRP	25
Blood film	No atypical lymphocytes
Throat swab	Negative

1. What is the most likely diagnosis?
    a   Kawasaki disease
    b   Follicular tonsillitis
    c   Glandular fever
    d   Adenovirus infection
    e   Viral hepatitis
    f   Tubercular lymphadenopathy
    g   Histocytosis
    h   Rubella virus infection
2. What one investigation is needed to confirm the diagnosis?
    a   Echocardiography
    b   Lymph node biopsy
    c   Mono spot test
    d   IgM for EBV
    e   ESR
    f   Skin biopsy
    g   Throat swab
    h   Repeat blood film

Case 38

A child aged 10 was admitted with right iliac fossa pain that was present for the last 24 hours, and has been getting worse over the last 3 hours. The surgeons raised the possibility of a UTI and the child was to be reviewed the next day. Analgesia and i.v. fluids were given and she was kept nil by mouth. Her abdominal pain got worse overnight and she was seen by a surgical senior house officer (SHO), who prescribed more analgesia (morphine). The paediatric team reviewed her in the morning, a diagnosis of appendicitis was made, and the surgeon agreed with this. She was operated on and a hemicolectomy was carried out due to adhesion following an appendicular mass. The ileocaecal part of the intestine is also involved. The test results are:

Hb	12.2 g/dl
WCC	15×10^9/l (N 70%)
PLT	560×10^9/l

| U&E | Normal |
| MSU | < 10 leukocytes and no organisms |

1. What are the most likely three differential diagnoses in order?
   a   Appendicitis
   b   Crohn's disease
   c   Intestinal tuberculosis
   d   Ileocaecal abscess
   e   Appendicular mass
   f   Perforated appendix
   g   Ulcerative colitis
2. Which two investigations will help to reach the diagnosis, in order?
   a   Immediate ESR
   b   Upper GIT endoscopy
   c   Mantoux test
   d   Histopathology of the surgical mass
   e   Lower GIT endoscopy
   f   Abdominal US
   g   Abdominal MRI

Case 39

A 5-month-old boy was admitted to a general paediatric ward with a history of jerking episodes in the last 10 days. Within 5–10 min of his going to sleep, his right arm starts jerking, with his fist clenching, and within a few seconds his left arm starts to do the same, which is followed by this type of movement in his legs. He never wakes up and there is no generalised tonic–clonic phase. His mother holds his arm or leg, but this does not stop the movement. On one occasion his face was involved; this lasted only a few seconds. The longest duration of these episodes was 3 min, but this was not continuous and could be interrupted by holding one of his limbs.

There were no other concerns about him; he smiled at the age of 7 weeks, has good head control and is able to roll from front to back. He sits with support and there are no concerns about his vision or hearing. He has no birthmarks and there is no history of epilepsy in the family. He has one sibling, aged 4, who is in good health.

He can smile with no facial asymmetry, follow objects without and problem and his eye movements are all normal. His power, tone and reflexes are all intact and equal in the upper and lower limbs. He is able to reach for an object without tremor or difficulties.

His asleep and awake EEG were reported as normal. Other test results are:

Hb	11.6 g/dl
WCC	7.2×10^9/l
PLT	250×10^9/l
Na	138 mmol/l

K	4.2 mmol/l
U	3.8mmol/l
Cr	44 mmol/l
ALT	38 IU/l
APH	126 IU/l
Alb	32 g/l
Glu	5.3 mmol/l
Lactate	2.1 mmol/l
NH_4	40 mmol/l

Venous gas at 10.00 p.m.

pH	7.38	pH	7.40 at 10.00 a.m.
PCO_2	2.4 kpa	PCO_2	4.5 kpa
PO_2	8.4 kpa	PO_2	9.6 kpa
HCO_3	14	HCO_3	16
Be	−13	Be	−0.3
Urine organic acid	Normal		
Serum AA	Normal		
Urine for reducing substances	Normal		
Cranial CT	No abnormalities		
Ketonuria	Negative		

1. What is the possible diagnosis?
   - a Benign neonatal familial convulsion
   - b Benign infantile convulsion
   - c Benign myoclonic epilepsy of infancy
   - d Infantile spasms
   - e Myoclonic astatic epilepsy
   - f Myoclonic encephalopathy
2. Which other tests may help the diagnosis?
   - a Cranial MRI
   - b Repeat sleep EEG
   - c Video telemetry
   - d Nothing
   - e Repeat metabolic screen
3. What treatment should be given?
   - a Vigabatrin
   - b Sodium valproate
   - c Lamotrigine
   - d Nothing
   - e Phenytoin

Case 40

An infant aged 11 months presented with a history of FTT. He is on solids and SMA Gold, up to a quantity of 600 ml/day. He likes boiled rice and pasta. He is not suffering from diarrhoea and has no rash. His father works long hours as a cook in a local Indian restaurant and his mother is a housewife. The whole family of nine live in a three-bedroomed terraced house. One of his older siblings was diagnosed with juvenile chronic arthritis (JCA), and is on treatment and responding very well. His sister, who is 11 years old, started her period 2 months ago and has been diagnosed as having mild anaemia. The parents are struggling to pay their mortgage.

His weight is 5.9 kg (on the 10th centile), his height is 84 cm (on the 25th centile) and his OFC is 45.6 cm (on the 50th centile).

No abnormalities are found upon systemic examination, but his nails are brittle and a pansystolic murmur can be heard on the left sternal border. Other test results are:

Hb	4.3 g/dl
WCC	$7.9 \times 10^9/l$ (N 45%, L 55%, E 1.3%)
PLT	$445 \times 10^9/l$
PCV	35 fl
Ret	1.4%
MCHC	19 g/dl
MCV	56 fl
Serum ferritin	1
IBC	30%

1. What are the three most likely diagnoses in order?
    a   Thalassaemia major
    b   Thalassaemia minor
    c   JCA
    d   Iron-deficiency anaemia
    e   Spherocytosis
    f   Lead poisoning
    g   Coeliac disease
    h   Crohn's disease
    i   Ulcerative colitis
    j   Cows' milk intolerance
2. What would you expect to see on the blood film, in order?
    a   Spherocytes
    b   Microcytosis
    c   Elliptocytosis
    d   Anisocytosis
    e   Target cells
    f   Basophilic stippling
    g   Howell–Jolly bodies
    h   Sideroblastic red cells
    i   Hypochromic red cells
    j   Spindle-shaped red cells

ANSWERS 31–40

Case 31

1. c   Normal
2. e   Lead level

3. a   Blood film
    c   Long-bone X-ray
4. Lead poisoning
5. b   Contact the Environmental Health Officer
    e   Start treatment again with strict supervision by the
        community care team

Chronic lead poisoning

This can occur after chewing or sucking lead paint from old
windows or doors. Lead from burning batteries, lead shot for
fishing, and old water pipes pose a similar risk. Children from
southeast Asia and the subcontinent may get lead poisoning from
using Surma, an eye make-up. They are usually known to have pica or
a compulsive eating disorder. They are usually anaemic and are
diagnosed as having iron deficiency anaemia and on treatment fail
to respond and the clinical situation changes. They will continue to
be anaemic, complain of abdominal pain, headache, and have
behavioural problems along with a deterioration in school
performance. Those with severe poisoning may present with
convulsions, irritability and unconsciousness, which may lead to coma
and death. The lead level can be measured and a blood film will show
hypochromic, microcytic red cells, and basophilic stippling. The long-
bone X-ray may show lead lines, which affect mainly the ends of the
long bones, and sometimes lead flakes may be seen on abdominal X-
ray. Lead poisoning is one of the causes of increased intracranial
pressure, and papilloedema is common. Removal of the child from the
affected environment as well as informing the Environmental Health
Officer is very important. Chelating agents can be used such as D-
penicillamine in mild cases and ethylenediaminetetraacetic acid
(EDTA) in severe cases. The effectiveness of EDTA can be enhanced by
giving dimercaprol as an i.m. injection.

Case 32

1. f   Abdominal US
    b   Hepatitis B serology
    c   Hepatitis C serology
    Blood film
2. On X-ray –   cupping, widening and flaring of epiphysis
                 osteopenia
    On photo –   rachitic rosary
3. a   Calcium
    b   Phosphorus
    c   Vitamin D level
    j   Parathyroid hormone level
    e   AAs
    h   Bone marrow aspiration
    f   Liver biopsy
4. Tyrosinaemia

Tyrosinaemia

This is one of the tyrosine metabolic disorders: tyrosinaemia type 1, tyrosinaemia type 2, alkaptonuria, and others. Tyrosinaemia leads to a high plasma level of tyrosine. In type 1, there will be hepatocellular damage, resulting in Fanconi syndrome. The affected person usually presents with FTT, profound rickets, thrombocytopenia and an abnormal clotting disorder. Hypertrophic cardiomyopathy may occur. There is an increased risk of hepatic carcinoma in patients who survive to adulthood. As a result there will be abnormal liver and kidney function, with a prolonged PT that will not respond to vitamin K. The plasma tyrosine and methionine levels are usually high. The serum alpha-fetoprotein level is very high and there is generalised aminoaciduria and tyrosyluria. Gamma-aminolevulinic acid excretion is increased. Neonates with hepatitis or older children with a family history of tyrosinaemia should be screened for this condition, especially if there is hepatocellular damage. Confirmation is by enzyme assay in cultured fibroblasts. A diet low in phenylalanine and tyrosine is important in these patients, but liver transplant surgery gives the only chance of survival in severe cases. NTBC is effective in reversing liver damage by reducing the level of succinylacetone to normal.

Case 33

1. g   CSA
    a   UTI
    d   Threadworms
    b   Valvovaginitis
2. c   Carry out a FME (urgently)
    b   Refer to Social Services
    g   Refer to child protection team

Child sexual abuse

Child sexual abuse was defined (Kempe 1978, p. 382) as the involvement of dependent, developmentally immature children and adolescents in sexual acts that they do not fully consent to, that they are not able to give informed consent for, or that violate the social taboos of family roles. A history of child sexual abuse is not uncommon among the general population, and the figure is as high as 38% in girls and 15% in boys. Females on average suffer sexual abuse significantly more often than males. The most common type of sexual abuse in males and females is fondling of the genital areas. The second most common form of sexual abuse of males involves the performance of oral sex, while abuse of females may vary from removal of clothing to direct genital contact. There is a strong association between physical and sexual abuse. One-third of physically abused children may be sexually abused and 12–15% of sexually abused children may be physically abused. The main perpetrators of sexual abuse of girls and boys are males who are acquaintances or strangers, rather than relatives. There should always be a high degree of suspicion in order to prevent sexual abuse cases in children. Each trust should have its own guidelines for dealing with children who are sexually abused and there are national guidelines as well. In cases in which doubt exists a second opinion should be sought, as many experts can help. Follow-up clinics, including the psychiatric genitourinary (GU) clinic and counselling, are very important.

Reference: Kempe X. 1987. Sexual abuse: another hidden paediatric problem. The 1977 C. Anderson Aldrich lectures. *Paediatrics* 62(3) 382–9.

Case 34

1. a   Immediate intubation and ventilation
   b   Give i.v. 10 ml/kg of 0.9% NaCl
   d   Start i.v. antibiotics (benzylpenicilllin and gentamicin)
   h   Echocardiography
2. f   No abnormalities
3. b   Hypothyroidism
   a   Sepsis

Hypothyroidism

This is the commonest treatable cause of mental retardation. It is a problem worldwide, and is most frequently due to iodine deficiency. Complete absence of thyroid tissue is the commonest cause of non-endemic hypothyroidism. The aetiology remains unknown in many cases but can be familial and associated with Down syndrome. Other causes of thyroid dyshormonogenesis include a decrease in TSH responsiveness and failure to concentrate iodide. The association of iodide organisation and sensorineural deafness is called Pendred syndrome. Not all thyroid dyshormonogenesis is associated with a loss of thyroid tissue, and in some cases the thyroid gland will be enlarged. TSH deficiency due to pituitary or hypothalamic abnormalities is a rare cause of hypothyroidism. Many classic features of hypothyroidism are not found in newborns. A large tongue, hoarse cry, facial puffiness, umbilical hernia, hypotonia, mottling, cold hands and feet, and lethargy are subtle and appear with time. There are non-specific signs that may suggest hypothyroidism, including unconjugated hyperbilirubinaemia, a gestation longer than 42 weeks, delayed passage of meconium and stool, respiratory distress, severe infection, feeding difficulties, and a large anterior fontanelle. Neonatal screening for hypothyroidism should be done at 1 week of age as earlier testing may reflect the mother's thyroid status and give a false-negative result. The diagnosis can be confirmed by a decrease in plasma T_4 and a rise in TSH of > 20 mU/l. Measurement of T_3 is of little value. A radionuclide scan will help to localise and measure the size of the gland. US of the neck will help to confirm the absence of the thyroid gland. Thyroid antibodies should be tested, as well as base-line cortisol, GH, LH and FSH. Replacement therapy with thyroxine (L-T_4) should start as soon as the diagnosis is confirmed. Genetic counselling is important and the prognosis is excellent.

Case 35

1. b   Cranial CT
   a   CXR
   f   Urine toxicology
2. a   Dilated lateral ventricles
3. c   Cranial MRI
   e   Mantoux test
   a   CSF for culture and sensitivity as well as PCR for
        Mycobacterium
4. e   Tubercular meningitis

Tubercular meningitis

Tubercular meningitis remains one of the leading causes of death in children. The number of cases of pulmonary tuberculosis has been increasing in recent years, and more cases occur in areas where sanitation is poor. Tuberculosis occurs first in the lungs and then spreads to the meninges, which may take 6 months. The symptoms are insidious and may take months to appear. The presenting symptoms are varied but there should be a high degree of suspicion in children who have been in contact with other patients with TB or who have travelled to highly endemic areas. Most often low-grade fever is present, followed by listlessness and irritability, which is mainly due to headache. Headache is the commonest feature; it is progressive and not alleviated by analgesia. Vomiting and abdominal pain may be associated with this condition. Headache and vomiting increase in frequency and the signs of meningitis appear later. Cerebral infarctions occur in 30–40% of cases. Seizures may appear early, but usually develop after meningism is established. The level of consciousness declines progressively, with focal neurological deficit. Papilloedema, cranial neuropathies and hemiparesis may follow, and death occurs if not treated early. The cause of hydrocephalus is the prevention of absorption of CSF by the choroid plexus due to deposits of infected material and a high content of protein in the CSF. The CSF will show a WCC of 100–250 cells/m^2 and predominant lymphocytes with low glucose and very high protein levels. AFB may be detected in the CSF but a culture will diagnose tubercular meningitis. A PCR study will help in diagnosing tubercular meningitis. Recovery is made by children who are not comatose at presentation. The mortality rate in some regions is as high as 20%.

Case 36

1. c   Half correction of acidosis with bicarbonate

h.v. 10 ml/kg of 0.9% NaCl over 30 min
2. f, h CO_2 high from acidosis correction or blocked ETT
3. Cerebral function monitoring (CFM)
4. Abnormal. There is evidence of seizure activity
5. b   Reload with phenobarbitone
   c   Maintenance with phenobarbitone
   g   Repeat cranial US
6. MACI
   Bright basal ganglia
   Internal capsule involvement
7. 10–15% chance of normal development
   e   Speech problem

Neonatal seizures

Neonatal seizures are poorly organised and difficult to recognise and distinguish from normal activity. They may arise from the brainstem or hemispheres. The possibility of seizures increases with brain abnormality. Seizures are usually accompanied by a change in HR, desaturation and an increase in systolic blood pressure. EEG may help to diagnose neonatal seizures. Video telemetry is the best way to diagnose neonatal seizures: marking the events on video and at the same time recording any EEG abnormalities. The epileptiform activity in newborns is usually widespread and can be detected even when the newborn is clinically asymptomatic.

The seizure patterns in newborns appear in different forms, which include:

- Apnoea with tonic stiffening of the body
- Focal clonic movements of one or both limbs on both sides
- Multifocal clonic limb movements
- Myoclonic jerks
- Paroxysmal laughing
- Tonic deviation of the eyes, upward or to one side
- Tonic stiffening of the body

The differential diagnosis of neonatal seizures is varied, but looking for treatable causes is very important. Rule out infection (bacterial or viral), electrolyte imbalance, IVH, cerebral haemorrhage, drugs, inborn errors of metabolism, HIE, cerebral dysgenesis and other brain abnormalities, familial neonatal seizures, and TS.

Stopping the seizures is important, but this depends on the cause. The administration of phenobarbitone or phenytoin as an infusion will help to stop seizures. It is very important to give maintenance therapy by administering these drugs via i.v. cannula and measuring levels to achieve an effective dose. Newborns who do not respond to phenobarbitone or phenytoin will require ventilation, and a clonazepam infusion will help to stop seizure activity. Muscle twitches can be stopped most of the time, but abnormal brain activity will continue and subsequently will either stop or evolve into another type of seizure with a different type of brain activity. Finding the cause is very important, as treatment with anticonvulsants will depend on finding the cause and treating this if it is treatable. The prognosis also depends on the cause.

Case 37

1. c   Glandular fever (infectious mononucleosis)
2. d   IgM for EBV

Glandular fever (infectious mononucleosis)

This is a disease of older children and young adults, and an almost identical clinical picture can be caused by CMV and *Toxoplasma gondii*. The initial presentation is usually not much different from that of any other URTI. It is characterised by fever, sore throat and enlarged cervical lymphadenopathy. It is associated with exudative tonsillitis. There are many complications that may be associated with this viral infection, including aseptic meningitis, transverse myelitis, and Bell's palsy and Guillain–Barré syndrome. Myocarditis, splenomegaly and a ruptured spleen are other complications, and patients should be warned against doing any contact sports if there is splenomegaly. Prolonged illnesses may cause fatigue, lethargy and frequent absence from school. The Paul–Bunnell test is a subjective test and the antibodies may take 2–3 weeks to develop. The specific EBV IgM antibody test is more readily available and is used to indicate current infection. The blood film will show atypical monocytes. There is no specific treatment and general advice for pain and temperature should be given. Children with chronic fatigue and lethargy should be helped at school and home. A multidisciplinary team including a psychologist, physiotherapist and paediatrician should work together to help the child as well as the family involved.

Case 38

1. e   Appendicular mass
    b   Crohn's disease
    d   Ileocaecal abscess
2. d   Histopathology of the surgical mass
    c   Mantoux test

Appendicitis

This is a very common condition in which diagnosis can be very difficult, and if in doubt surgery is advised. An emergency surgical procedure is needed, as if left untreated, the appendix may perforate and cause many problems, or may cause the development of an appendicular mass that may resemble Crohn's disease. This is still a condition with a significant rate of mortality and morbidity. It usually presents with abdominal pain, fever and vomiting. The abdominal pain is usually periumbilical and radiates to the right iliac fossa. The child will have a coated tongue, be restless because of the pain, will not be able to walk upright and will find it very difficult to climb up onto the table for examination. There will be tenderness, guarding, and rebound phenomena will be positive at examination of the right iliac fossa. No single blood or radiological test will diagnose appendicitis; they can help but every case can present differently. There should always be a high index of suspicion, and surgery should not be delayed as the rate of morbidity is high in patients with a perforated appendix. US is helpful in recognising a thickened appendix with surrounding oedema. The differential diagnosis of an appendicular mass can include ileocaecal tuberculosis, Crohn's disease and terminal ileitis. Conditions associated with appendicitis include mesenteric adenitis, gastroenteritis, constipation, torsion ovarian cyst, Meckel's diverticulitis, salpingitis, UTI, right basal pneumonia, Henoch–Schönlein purpura, diabetes mellitus and sickle-cell crisis.

Case 39

1. c   Benign myoclonic epilepsy of infancy
2. b   Repeat sleep EEG
3. d   Nothing

Benign myoclonic epilepsy of infancy

This condition is very rare and occurs in infants between the ages of 4 months and 3 years. As the child falls asleep and within 10–30 min, generalised myoclonic jerks of the limbs will occur, which may be repeated several times. It will not affect sleep or cause the child to wake up. The jerks will not stop if someone holds the child's hand and can be felt. The EEG is usually normal, but may show generalised spikes or polyspikes during the interictal phase. This condition is usually idiopathic. No further tests or treatment are required in most cases, unless it causes problems or anxiety in the family, and in this case drugs may help. The prognosis is very good and it is very rare for this condition to develop to generalised tonic–clonic seizures or affect the development of the child.

Case 40

1. d   Iron-deficiency anaemia
    h   Crohn's disease
    g   Coeliac disease
2. b   Microcytosis
    i   Hypochromic red cells
    d   Anisocytosis

Iron-deficiency anaemia

This is one of the commonest types of anaemia, affecting children in inner cities more than in rural areas. Poor nutrition and diet play a large part in causing this in children. Poverty and social problems are cofactors, when healthy food is not affordable. Other causes of iron-deficiency anaemia are impaired iron absorption and excessive loss of iron due to bleeding. Infestation with worms is one of the commonest causes of iron-deficiency anaemia worldwide. Chronic blood loss from the gut due to inflammation secondary to inflammatory bowel disease or chronic infection will lead to iron-deficiency anaemia. Any chronic blood loss from any part of the body will lead to iron-deficiency anaemia. The affected child will look pale and tired, and this will affect their performance in school. Looking for a cause is important. Dietary intake and nutritional history for all family members is very important. When iron supplementation is started for treatment of iron-deficiency anaemia secondary to insufficient dietary intake, all family members should receive the supplement, and support from the dietitian, health visitor and if necessary a social worker is needed. Oral treatment is the starting point of treatment, and if there is poor compliance and no other cause can be found, i.v. treatment should be considered, although this is rarely needed. Recovery is usually very good, especially for children attending school.

Case 41

A mother brought her 4-week-old boy to A&E, as he was irritable and febrile. He was seen 2 weeks previously, with a history of rash, which was diagnosed as seborrhoeic dermatitis. He was a full-term normal delivery (FTND) and has had no difficulties in the first 2 weeks of life. He is the first child born to healthy parents and there is no family history of illness. He was admitted and a full septic screen was carried out. Two hours after admission he started having tonic–clonic seizures in his left arm, which lasted for 2 min; this happened about three times. He was given a loading dose of phenobarbitone and he continued to have focal seizures, which required another half loading dose of phenobarbitone. His seizures became more generalised tonic–clonic seizures and he was transferred to a specialist centre for further management. He was intubated and paralysed to control seizures. The test results are:

Na	134 mmol/l
K	4.3 mmol/l
U	4.1 mmol/l
Ca	2.44 mmol/l
Mg	0.99 mmol/l
Glu	5.8 mmol/l
Bilirubin	42 μmol/l
Urine pH	6
RAS	Negative
ALT	24 IU/l
Alb	38 g/l
CRP	< 5
ESR	< 2 mm/hour
MSU	Negative
Stool	No growth
CXR	Normal
Cranial CT	No abnormalities
Hb	14.2 g/dl
WCC	17.2×10^9/l (L 7.4, N 6.1)
PLT	459×10^9/l
PTT	39 s
TT	1 s
INR	1.3

CSF

WCC	100 (75% lymphocytes)
RBC	15
Protein	0.99 g/l
Glu	2.4 mmol/l
No organism	
Serum glu	4.5 mmol/l
NH_3	28 mmol/l

Lactate	1.8 mmol/l
pH	7.38
PCO_2	5.2 kpa
PO_2	8.3 kpa
Be	−0.2
Urine pH	**6**

1. What is the most likely diagnosis?
   - a   Viral meningitis
   - b   Bacterial meningitis
   - c   Viral encephalitis
   - d   Herpes encephalitis
   - e   Tubercular meningitis
   - f   Metabolic encephalopathy
   - g   Non-accidental injury
   - h   HIV
   - i   Toxic encephalopathy
2. Which first three lines of drugs should be used in this case?
   - a   Cefotaxime or ceftriaxone
   - b   Gentamicin
   - c   Benzylpenicillin
   - d   Erythromycin
   - e   Aciclovir
   - f   Metronidazole
   - g   Rifampicin
   - h   Streptomycin
   - i   Ganciclovir
3. Which other two tests should the laboratory carry out on the sample of CSF?
   - a   PCR for viruses (HSV, EBV, adenovirus)
   - b   PCR for bacteria (*Neisseria*, *Pneumococcus*, and *Haemophilus influenzae*)
   - c   Culture
   - d   *Mycoplasma* titres
   - e   Oligoclonal bands
   - f   Lactate
   - g   Pyruvate
   - h   Glycine
   - i   Zeil Gram stain

Case 42

A 13-year-old boy presented with a history of absence attacks since the age of 9 years; these start as staring with his eyes fluttering in episodes of 5–10 s duration, and then he returns to normal. He may have up to 100 of these attacks per day. He was an FTND and there are no concerns about his development. He is doing well at school. The results of the general and systemic examinations were normal. The awake EEG was reported as normal on two occasions. He was treated with sodium valproate but developed a behavioural problem, becoming aggressive and violent with other children. At the moment he is taking lamotrigine and ethosuximide, which are not helping him. In the last 2 months, he has had three generalised tonic–clonic seizures in the morning. His mother said that he had no jerks on these occasions but he said that sometimes when he is doing something requiring concentration he does have jerks (and also sometimes in the morning). There is a problem with his complying with medication.

1. What is the most likely diagnosis?
   a   Atypical absence seizures
   b   Absence epilepsy
   c   Juvenile myoclonic epilepsy
   d   Generalised tonic–clonic epilepsy on awakening
   e   Absence with eye myoclonia
   f   Benign Rolandic epilepsy of childhood
   g   Juvenile absence epilepsy
2. What abnormalities appear on this EEG?

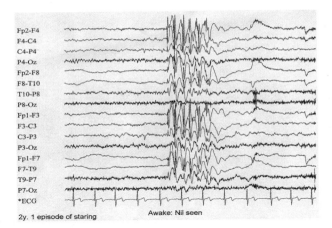

2y. 1 episode of staring   Awake: Nil seen

   a   Generalised spike and wave of 3 Hz/s
   b   Generalised spike and wave of 4 Hz/s with photosensitivity
   c   Polyspikes and waves with 4–5 Hz/s
   d   Generalised polyspike and waves
3. Which other anticonvulsants, in order, should be tried for controlling his seizures?
   a   Carbamazepine
   b   Topiramate
   c   Levatricetam
   d   Oxycarbamazepine
   e   Sodium valproate

f   Vigabatrin
g   Clonazepam
h   Clobazam

Case 43

A 5-year-old child presented with a history of diarrhoea and
vomiting in the last 3 days. His vomiting is less frequent now but his
diarrhoea is getting worse and his mother described his stool
form as 'runny and smelly'. He had the same symptoms 3 months
ago, which resolved within 3 days and no cause was found on stool
culture. He is not interested in any food other than sweets and
biscuits. He has been complaining of a sharp pain in the right iliac
fossa, which lasts for 1–2 hours and then disappears. He was
swimming in the sea 2 weeks ago with his brother and father. The
upper GIT endoscopy and biopsy show partial villous atrophy. The
coeliac screen and test for lactose milk intolerance were negative.
Other test results are:

Hb	7.3 g/dl
WCC	15.6 × 10⁹/l (N 6.3, L 3.0, E 2.1)
PLT	425 × 10⁹/l
CRP	20
ESR	2 mm/hour
LFT	Normal
Abdominal US	Normal
Stool	A lot of mucus and blood
MSU	15 white cells only and C/S no growth

1.   What is the most likely diagnosis?
2.   Which other three tests should be carried out?

Case 44

On her 13th birthday, a girl presented to A&E with a history of a
reduced level of consciousness and lethargy. She was out all day with
her mother, and after she returned home, she felt unwell, went to
sleep and her mother found her difficult to rouse. She has been
unwell in the past few months, with abdominal pain that was
diagnosed as constipation. She looks pale and skinny. Her aunt died
of hepatic failure at the age of 44 years. There is no consanguinity.
Her sister is 7 years old, fit and well apart from one vaginal bleed last
week. The girl responds to pain but does not open her eyes. Her
serum glucose level is 2.4 mmol/l and her BP is 65/50 mmHg. Her
temperature is 36.8°C, her HR is 110/min and capillary refill time (CRT)
is 4 s centrally.

1.   What should be the initial management of this case?
     a   Resuscitation fluid
     b   Secure airway

    c   Ventilate
    d   Give antibiotics
    e   Give antiviral agent
    f   Urine for toxicology
    g   Transfer to ITU
    h   Ask for help
    i   Send blood for FBC, U&E, LFT, clotting, culture, blood group
         and safe

The girl was resuscitated and the blood results came back. She was transferred to the liver unit, ventilated for 7 days and put on a waiting list for a liver transplant. She developed abnormal movement in her upper limbs. The test results are:

Hb	7.2 g/dl
WWC	$4.3 \times 10^9/l$
PLT	$120 \times 10^9/l$
INR	6
PTT	> 100 s
PT	> 30 s
ALT	320 IU/l
ALP	2250 IU/l
Alb	16 g/l
Na	126 mmol/l
K	5.3 mmol/l
Ca	1.88 mmol/l
Mg	0.66 mmol/l

2. What are the differential diagnoses and in what order?
    a   Renal failure
    b   Septicaemia
    c   Intoxication
    d   Hepatic failure
    e   Metabolic disorders
    f   Hepatitis
    g   Encephalopathy
    h   Heavy metal poisoning
3. Which other three tests should you carry out and what order?
    a   Blood culture
    b   Urine toxicology
    c   CRP
    d   Urinary copper
    e   Caeruloplasmin
    f   Blood gas
    g   Viral serology
    h   LP
    i   Abdominal US
    j   Cranial MRI
    k   Liver biopsy

4. What is/are the abnormality/ies on this photo?

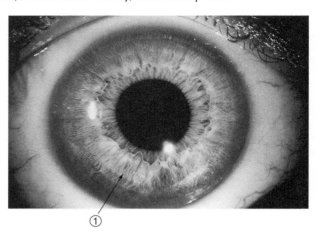

Case 45

A father accompanied his 14-year-old daughter to a children's outpatient department and she was seen by a GP. She had a UTI, was feeling lethargic and had double vision. She was referred to hospital for a second opinion. She always feels tired, especially at weekends and at the end of the day. She was well before and has no previous history of eye problems. Her family has no history of eye problems. She plays hockey at school and is also a keen cyclist. Her family lives in a four-bedroomed house, with one cat. Both parents are teachers and she has two brothers, who are healthy. She looks tired, has both eyes half-closed and she finds it difficult to open her eyes; she has to tilt her head backward to be able to look to someone. Her eye movement is intact; her pupils react equally and she has no problem with her visual field. Her fundi are very easily visualised and there is no evidence of papilloedema. Her other cranial nerves are all intact. She said she feels weak in her body but her reflexes are all present; she can lift her arms and legs against gravity, with normal tone. She feels stronger in her lower limbs than in her upper limbs. She was admitted to hospital for further testing, and in the evening she choked on her food and found it difficult to breathe. She was given 10 L/min oxygen via a facemask, which helped a little. By midnight she was intubated and transferred to the PICU. Her CXR was normal and blood gas testing showed respiratory acidosis. Her EEG and cranial MRI with contrast showed no abnormalities. An LP carried out in the PICU was reported to be normal. Lactate, ammonia, AAs and organic acids were reported to be normal. She continued on a ventilator for 7 days and made a good recovery with treatment.

1. What is the most likely diagnosis?
    a   Viral encephalitis
    b   ADEM

c   Intoxication
d   Myasthenia gravis
e   Myotonic dystrophy
f   Dermatomyositis
g   Myeloencephalitis
h   Inborn error of metabolism
i   Midbrain astrocytoma
j   Meningitis
k   Guillain–Barré syndrome
2.   Which three investigations are required to prove your diagnosis?

Case 46

A 7-year-old boy presented with a history of malaise, poor weight
gain and a large spleen. He had an operation in the first 5 weeks of
life to correct biliary atresia. The operation was successful and he
was discharged from follow-up at the age of 2 years, fit and well. He
has been well since, apart from viral infections and one admission to
hospital with jaundice at the age of 4, which resolved completely;
various blood tests and abdominal US showed no abnormalities
apart from a raised ALT level, which at that time was ignored as it
was considered to be not significant. In the past 6 weeks he has been
feeling unwell, with lethargy, non-specific muscle pain, abdominal
pain and headaches. His doctor examined him 2 weeks ago and
found that he had a large spleen and distended abdomen. He was
referred for an abdominal X-ray, which did not show anything apart
from a large spleen. When he was seen in the clinic, he was
lethargic, pale and said his energy is gone. He sleeps a lot, his
appetite is reduced and he has started losing weight. His spleen
measures about 4 cm below the left costal margin, with smooth
edges and is mildly tender, and there is no organomegaly. An
abdominal US showed a spleen measuring 5–6 cm, a liver
measuring 3 cm below the costal margin and polycystic kidneys.
The test results are:

Hb	8.2 g/dl
WCC	$2.1 \times 10^9/l$ (N 60%)
PLT	$100 \times 10^9/l$
Na	135 mmol/l
K	4.2 mmol/l
Alb	26 g/l
Total protein	55 g/l
ALT	166 IU/l
γGT	150 IU/l
Bilirubin	20 μmol/l
INR	1.3
PTT	55 s
PT	12 s
HBsA	Negative
HBsAg	Negative

HBC	Negative
Blood film	Target cells
AlK. Ph	360 IU/l
ANA	Negative

1.   What is the most likely diagnosis?
2.   Which other two tests should be carried out?
3.   What is the prognosis?

Case 47

An 11-year-old boy presented to A&E with a history of diarrhoea and vomiting in the last 24 hours. He was at school the day before and was sent home, as he felt unwell and had abdominal pain. He said he has been feeling unwell for the last 4 weeks, with generalised weakness and lethargy. His friends commented that his skin is suntanned, even though he has not been on holiday for the last 2 years. He was a FTND. He had viral meningitis when he was 7 years old but recovered well. His father was diagnosed as having irritable bowel syndrome 3 years ago. His mother has chronic asthma. His younger brother and sister are healthy. He likes dogs and was promised a dog if he passed his GCSE exams.

He looks darker than his brother, his BP is 95/55 mmHg, and his HR 80 b.p.m. There is no evidence of skin lesions and his abdomen is generally tender but soft, with active bowel sounds. The test results are:

Na	128 mmol/l
K	6.2 mmol/l
Ur	12.2 mmol/l
Cr	77 mmol/l
ALT	38 IU/l
AlK. Ph	125 IU/l
Alb	27 g/l
Hb	9.8 g/dl
WCC	7.3×10^9/l (N 10%, L 80%)
PLT	180×10^9/l
MSU	Ketones positive
BS	2.5 mmol/l
Stool	No blood and C/S is negative
Abdominal US	Normal
Ca	2.90 mmol/l
HCO_3	13 mmol/l

1.   What is the most likely diagnosis?
    a   Septicaemia
    b   Chronic renal failure
    c   Metabolic disorder
    d   Addisonian crisis
    e   Wilson's disease
    f   Lead poisoning
    g   Chronic liver disease

    h   Acute porphyries
2. What are the four most significant tests that should be carried
    out?
    a   Urinary copper
    b   Urinary coproporphyrin
    c   Lead level
    d   Midnight cortisol level
    e   Urinary hydroxyprogesterone or steroid level
    f   Blood gas
    g   Hepatitis B and C serology
    h   Renal US
    i   GFR
    j   Serum AAs
    k   Lactate level
    l   Urine toxicology
    m   Short Synacthen test
    n   Abdominal MRI
3. What should the management plan be in three steps?
    a   I.v. antibiotics
    b   Daily glucocorticoid
    c   Daily mineralocorticosteroid replacement therapy
    d   Haemodialysis
    e   Detoxication with DTA
    f   Liver transplant
    g   Renal transplant
    h   Full endocrine work-up
    i   Cranial MRI

Case 48

A mother brought her daughter for the second time in the last 24
hours to A&E, with abdominal pain and frequent passing of a soft
stool in the last 2 days. The 4-year-old was fit and well before this
illness. She was sent home after she was assessed at hospital; she is
not dehydrated and does not look septic. Two days later she
presented with similar symptoms: headache, lethargy, more
abdominal pain, malaise and a pain in her neck. Her mother said her
temperature is going up every day, and today reached 40°C for the
first time. She also developed erythematous papular lesions, which
measure about 2 mm in diameter. All members of her family are
healthy and returned from a Mediterranean cruise holiday 6 days ago.
There is a 2 cm splenomegaly, with no lymphadenopathy. Her HR is
77 b.p.m., her RR/20 min, and her CRT < 2 s.

Na	130 mmol/l
K	3.9 mmol/l
Ur	8.3 mmol/l
Cr	76 mmol/l
ALT	55 IU/l
Alk. Ph	290 IU/l

Bilirubin	35 μmol/l
Hb	11.3g/dl
WCC	2.2×10^9/l (L 66%, N 22%)
PLT	90×10^9/l
MSU	Negative
Stool	Negative
Abdominal US	Large spleen only

1. What is the most likely diagnosis?
2. Which two other tests are required to support the diagnosis?
3. What should the treatment be in this case, in three steps?

Case 49

A 10-year-old boy presented with a history of right limb pain, which is getting worse. He was playing football at school this morning with other children. He fell a few times but had no bruises or cuts on his limbs. He had limb pain on and off in 7 of the last 12 hours but it was not as extreme as he currently feels. He had had no joint swelling or rashes associated with this pain before. No one in his family suffers from a joint or bone problem. He said he could not walk after he got back from school. He has a low-grade temperature and is not able to bear weight on his feet. His left lower limb is difficult to move. He can bend his knees up to 90° on the right but only up to 70° on the left. He can do full hip flexion, abduction and internal rotation on the right side, but finds it very difficult to do it on the left side. He has a generalised tenderness on his upper thigh and keeps his left lower limb in a flexion position at the hip and knee joints.

Hb	14.2 g/dl
WCC	14.3×10^9/l (N 75%)
PLT	350×10^9/l
CRP	20
ESR	12 mm/hour

1. Which other tests, in order, should be carried out immediately?
    a   X-ray of hips and knees
    b   US of hips
    c   Abdominal US
    d   Blood culture
    e   Urine for VMA
    f   Bone scan
    g   MRI of both lower limbs
    h   CT scan of lower limbs
    i   Hip aspiration
2. What two abnormalities appear on this hip X-ray?
    a   Dislodged left femoral epiphysis
    b   Reduced joint space on left
    c   Reduced bone density on the left
    d   Fragmentation of femoral head on the left
    e   Swollen soft tissues around the left hip joints

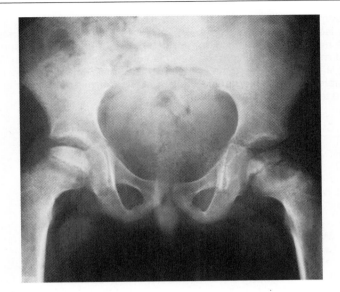

3. What is the most likely diagnosis?
   a Perthes' disease
   b JCA
   c Septic arthritis
   d Osteomyelitis
   e Slipped femoral epiphysis
   f Neuroblastoma
   g Osteosarcoma
   h TB arthritis

Case 50

A toddler, aged 2 years, was referred by her doctor for fresh bruises on her face. Her childminder looked after her all day. Only that morning her father had been working from home and left home for a business trip before lunchtime. The mother said that her daughter woke up at 3.00 p.m. with the bruises on her face. Her childminder said that the bruises were not there before the child's afternoon sleep, and that since the morning, she was clingy, wanted to go with her mother, refused to have her breakfast, and felt hot at that time. She played outside with her older brother, who is 3 years old, for about 2 hours. Her mother is working full time as a director of advertising in a family company. There were no other concerns and the childminder looked after the mother's children for the last 3 years. They visited a farmhouse 2 days ago and the children played with the animals and spent all day at the farm. The girl looks tired, her temperature is 37.5°C and her HR is 90 b.p.m.; there were no other abnormalities found on examination apart from a red throat. The bruises are about 5 cm long and about three of them are located on the right side of her face, anterior to her right ear. There is another red mark, which is 1 cm long and is located on her right shin. There are a few petechial rashes on her right fronto-parietal region, not visible on the skin, but can be seen at the margin of the hair and skin. The test results are:

HB	13.2 g/dl
WCC	$8.2 \times 10^9/l$ (L 60%)
PLT	$240 \times 10^9/l$
INR	1
PTT	35 s
PT	10 s
LFT & U&E	Normal
MSU	Negative
CRP	< 10

1. What is the diagnosis?
   a Trauma injuries
   b Viral infection
   c Slapped-cheek disease
   d Glandular fever
   e Streptococcal septicaemia
   f Sunburn
   g NAI
2. List, in order, four steps required for her management?
   a Admit the child and inform the duty consultant
   b Viral serology
   c Start i.v. antibiotics
   d Inform Social Services and the Child Protection Team
   e Check child protection register
   f Discharge home
   g Give prophylactic antibiotics to all family members in contact with the child in the last 24 hours
   h Arrange for photos and skeletal survey
   i Inform the microbiologist
   j Arrange for photography
   k Transfer to specialist unit
   l Tell parents about your concerns

ANSWERS 41–50

Case 41

1. c Viral encephalitis
2. d Erythromycin
   a Cefotaxime or ceftriaxone
   e Aciclovir

3. a   PCR for viruses (HSV, EBV, adenovirus)
    d   *Mycoplasma* titres

Viral encephalitis

Acute presentation with fever, headache, lethargy, nausea, and vomiting should alert the attending doctor to consider a diagnosis of encephalitis as the first choice. There is a high incidence of focal neurology associated with the presentation of encephalitis, especially with herpes simplex encephalitis. Older children with encephalitis usually complain of headache and will have behavioural changes: one minute they are OK, talking and doing things, and the next minute they will have bizarre behaviour and be confused. One of the commonest focal neurology signs is seizures, which are almost always focal, then become generalised. Other neurological signs such as those associated with meningitis will be very rare. A high degree of clinical suspicion will prompt immediate cover for herpes simplex, *Mycoplasma* and bacterial infection. Investigation, which includes LP, is important if the child is stable. EEG is helpful when available, but not necessary. Cranial CT is important, with contrast, as it may show some changes. The course of treatment depends on the findings from CSF and blood. If herpes simplex encephalitis is present, then a minimum of 3 weeks' i.v. treatment is recommended and recurrence is possible after stopping the treatment. For other viruses it is not yet known which antiviral is best, and consultation with a virologist is important.

Case 42

1. c   Juvenile myoclonic epilepsy
2. b   Generalised spike and wave of 4 Hz/s with photosensitivity
3. e   Sodium valproate
    b   Topiramate
    h   Clobazam

Juvenile myoclonic epilepsy

Clumsiness occurs in the morning, soon after the affected individual wakes up. It is usually familial and the age of onset is between 12 and 18 years in the majority of patients. The myoclonus is usually brief, bilateral and consists of flexor jerks of the arms, which may occur many times. If there are no generalised tonic–clonic seizures, consciousness will be retained. Generalised tonic–clonic seizures may occur as a result of sleep deprivation, alcohol intake and awakening from nocturnal or day sleep. This condition is associated with generalised tonic–clonic and absence seizures. Seizures are usually associated with polyspike and slow waves on the awake EEG. The polyspike discharges are also concurrent with seizures in ictal recording. Seizures are sometimes precipitated by photic stimulation or eye closure. They are exacerbated by carbamazepine and phenytoin, and thus these drugs should be avoided at all times. The drugs of choice should be sodium valproate and lamotrigine. Life-long treatment is required, should not be stopped and very rarely high doses are needed. Some children are not controlled on monotherapy, especially patients with generalised tonic–clonic seizures, and may require a second drug.

Case 43

1. Giardiasis
2. Repeat stool analysis (three warm samples)
   Immunoglobulins

Giardiasis

Giardiasis is caused by parasitic infection (*Giardia lamblia*). There are two stages: the first is the atrophozoite, which infests the proximal small intestine in children. Significant mucosal damage occurs, usually partial villous atrophy, but sometimes to the flat mucosa. The other form is an oval cyst, which can survive in soil and water for several months; it is the most infective form, even from person to person. Immune deficiency, malnutrition and hypoacidity are the predisposing factors to infection with the *G. lamblia* cyst. There is either a carrier state or an acute diarrhoeal illness, or chronic diarrhoea and intestinal malabsorption. Most children fall into the carrier category. Children with FTT and chronic or intermittent diarrhoea should be investigated for this parasitic infection. Stool culture and microscopic examination will diagnose infection with *G. lamblia*. Multiple stool samples are required if other causes of chronic diarrhoea cannot be found, and there should be a high degree of suspicion of giardiasis. Occasionally intestinal biopsy may reveal the parasitic infection. Metronidazole is the drug of choice and should be administered for 10 days. For immunocompromised patients, this drug may need to be administered for up to 6 weeks.

Case 44

1. h   Ask for help
   b   Secure airway
   f   Urine for toxicology
   d, e Give antibiotics and antiviral agent
   g   Transfer to ITU
   i   Send blood for FBC,U&E, LFT, clotting, culture, blood group
        and save serum
2. e   Metabolic disorders
   d   Hepatic failure
   c   Intoxication
   g   Encephalopathy
3. e   Caeruloplasmin
   d   Urinary copper

    k   Liver biopsy

4.   Kayser–Fleischer ring

Wilson's disease (hepatolenticular degeneration)

This disease is inherited as an autosomal recessive disorder and caused by a disturbance in the biliary excretion of copper and its incorporation into caeruloplasmin. The defective gene is located on chromosome 13 and symptoms are caused by deposition of copper in the brain, liver and cornea. The commonest presentation in children is hepatic failure, usually without neurological manifestation. Neurological manifestations occur in the second decade, with minimal liver problems. The initial symptoms are disturbances in gait or speech, and may remain unchanged for years. Other symptoms will appear and the initial symptoms will worsen. New symptoms include dysarthria, dystonia, rigidity, gait and postural abnormalities, tremor, and drooling. This disease is also associated with psychiatric symptoms prior to the appearance of neurological symptoms, such as behavioural disturbance, paranoid psychoses, and dementia later on. The corneal features in the form of Kayser–Fleischer rings will be certain features of the disease; this is caused by the deposition of copper in the Descemet's membrane and is present in almost all of these patients. Wilson's disease should be considered in children with dystonia and dysarthria, and in those with any chronic liver disease. The caeruloplasmin level will be reduced to less than 20 mg/l. Cranial MRI will demonstrate increased signal intensity and decreased size of the caudate, putamen, subcortical white matter, midbrain, and pons. The treatment of choice is oral D-penicillamine and is not to be discontinued. Genetic counselling for other members of the family is important.

Case 45

1.   d   Myasthenia gravis
2.   Edrophonium test
      Anti-acetylcholine receptor antibodies
      EMG

Myasthenia gravis

This is a disease of the neuromuscular junction, and is characterised by proximal muscle weakness and increased fatiguability on muscular exercise. It can be a congenital, autoimmune disease of neuromuscular blockage due to toxins or drugs. In autoimmune cases, it usually starts after 1 year of age and is more prevalent in adolescent girls. The onset is usually insidious, with involvement of the extraocular muscles with unilateral or bilateral ophthalmoplegia and/or ptosis. This will be followed by involvement of the proximal and bulbar muscles, which may lead to difficulty in swallowing. In some cases it may take weeks and months to spread from the ocular muscles to other muscles. This weakness is variable. Many patients may only complain of increasing fatigue. They feel normal on awakening, but as the day passes, they feel more fatigued and weak, especially following exercise. Examination will show normal reflexes and weakness in the proximal muscle group. There will be bilateral ptosis with a history of double vision. The EMG will show abnormal repetitive stimulation and will help in diagnosis. Abnormalities will be identified by the edrophonium chloride (Tensilon) test. In 60–80% of patients, the presence of antibodies against acetylcholine receptors will be shown. The creatinine kinase level is normal and muscle biopsy will show no specific features. The diagnosis can be confirmed by the Tensilon test. The test should be carried out in hospital with resuscitation equipment ready, in case the child becomes hypoxic or develops respiratory arrest. The child should have a testing dose and the full dose should be given after 30 s. Video camera footage or photos should be taken in order to observe the changes. An anticholinesterase agent will be very helpful. This is life-long treatment and in some patients other treatments such as corticosteroids or azathioprine can be used. Thymectomy can be considered for patients when medication is not helpful. Plasmapheresis can be performed in acute situations, when drugs have not had much effect and the child's general condition is deteriorating, but its use is very limited.

Case 46

1. Portal hypertension secondary to hepatic cirrhosis
2. Cholangiography
   ERCP
3. Poor without liver transplantation

Cirrhosis of the liver

In a cirrhotic liver there is replacement of normal liver tissue with nodules of liver cells that are growing in an unorganised fashion with too much fibrous tissue. Portosystemic shunts are present due to abnormal anastomosis, resulting from abnormal derangement of liver cells and tissues. As a consequence there will be abnormal liver function and portal hypertension will arise. There are many causes, which can be classified as genetic, biliary, postnecrotic and venous congestion. Liver biopsy is very important in finding the cause. Management should be directed to the cause. Before a biopsy is carried out, any clotting problem should be corrected, and a biopsy from the affected tissue for biochemical, immunological and DNA studies is important. Children with cirrhosis of the liver will achieve some growth in the first few years with structured management. The diet should contain sufficient protein, essential fatty acids, minerals, trace elements and vitamins, and the caloric intake should be at least 40% above the normal requirement. If hepatic failure arises, then the amount of protein should be reduced or stopped. Portal hypertension will cause splenomegaly, ascites and a growth problem. A large spleen will cause much discomfort. Ascites, if mild, can be treated with spironolactone and, if severe, frusemide can be added. The ultimate goal for cirrhosis of the liver is liver transplantation. Palpable kidneys occur in multipolycystic kidney disease, which has no relation to cirrhosis of the liver.

Case 47

1. Addisonian crisis
2. Abdominal MRI
   Low-dose dexamethasone-suppression test
   Midnight cortisol level
   Short Synacthen test
3. Daily glucocorticoid-replacement therapy
   Daily mineralocorticoid-replacement therapy
   Cranial MRI

Acute primary adrenal insufficiency (Addisonian crisis)

Acute adrenal insufficiency occurs in children with undiagnosed chronic adrenal insufficiency. These children, when exposed to additional stress such as with major illness, trauma or surgery, may suffer an acute adrenal crisis. They may present with signs of shock and abdominal pain, fever, hypoglycaemia, seizures, weakness (mainly proximal), apathy, vomiting, nausea, hyponatraemia, hyperkalaemia, metabolic acidosis, hypochloraemia, hypotension, and tachycardia, which may lead to cardiopulmonary collapse and death if not recognised and treated. Fluid replacement is important, as well as an ample dose of glucocorticoid with the aim being long-term treatment with glucocorticoids and mineralocorticoids. Adrenal crisis may follow from massive adrenal haemorrhage in a newborn who has lost a lot of blood during birth. There will be a palpable flank mass and microscopic haematuria. US is very good at identifying the mass and abdominal CT is also helpful. Adrenal crises can occur with meningococcal septicaemia as well (Waterhouse–Friderichsen syndrome). There will be a massive adrenal haemorrhage, and it may also be associated with septicaemia secondary to streptococcus, pneumococcus or diphtheria.

Primary adrenocortical insufficiency is due to destruction of the adrenal cortex, reducing production of gluco-mineralocorticoid and sex steroids. It is usually an autoimmune disease and can be associated with *HLA-DR3* and *HLA-B8*. Symptoms include weakness, anorexia, malaise, postural hypotension, abdominal symptoms, myalgia and arthralgia, hyperpigmentation, and neuropsychiatric manifestations. Addisonian crisis is characterised by the rapid onset of hypotension, tachycardia, fever, hypoglycaemia and deteriorating mental status. Biochemical changes occur in the majority of patients and include hyponatraemia, hyperkalaemia, raised urea level, hypoglycaemia, hypercalcaemia, and metabolic and respiratory acidosis. Other features include normocytic anaemia and leucopenia.

Random measurement of cortisol is often unhelpful, but the short Synacthen test can be helpful in diagnosing the disease. It is also associated with positive autoantibodies in 60–70% of affected individuals. Replacement therapy is with glucocorticoids and mineralocorticoids, but looking for the cause is vital and the prognosis is dependent on the cause of the Addison's disease. Children in whom Addisonian crisis is suspected on first presentation should be investigated fully for an underlying endocrine problem.

Case 48

1. Typhoid fever
2. Repeat stool culture
    Salmonella typhi serology (O & H antibodies)
3. I.v. fluids
    Antibiotics (ciproflucloxacillin)
    Hygiene

Typhoid fever

S. typhi only infects humans, and causes typhoid fever when an individual eats contaminated food. *S. typhi* can survive for a long time, even in frozen or dried food. After an incubation period of usually 10–14 days, vague influenza-like illness with fever, malaise, pains and headache develops. The fever persists for a week and the child will become ill with vomiting, abdominal pain, diarrhoea and cough. There will sometimes be constipation in older children. The affected child looks septic and confused, and has a high temperature. There will be tachycardia and tachypnoea, but later on, as the disease progresses, bradycardia may evolve and chest signs will appear. There is generalised tenderness in the abdomen, which is also distended. There may be meningeal signs and hepatosplenomegaly in many cases. Sometimes perforation of the gut may occur, especially in the second or third week of illness. This is usually associated with sudden deterioration, hypotension, tachycardia, abdominal pain and rigidity. The blood culture is positive in more than two-thirds of patients in the first week, but only in half of these patients will the stool sample be positive. The Widal test may be helpful; an O antibody of more than four-fold will indicate infection with *S. typhi* but a high H antibody will indicate previous infection or vaccination. Anaemia, hyponatraemia and thrombocytopenia occur with this illness. Supportive treatment with careful electrolytes and fluid balance is more important than trying to treat the infection with antibiotics. Chloramphenicol, co-trimoxazole and amoxicillin are very effective in treating *S. typhi*. Ceftriaxone and ciproflucloxacillin are used more frequently these days as species of *S. typhi* become more resistant to other antibiotics. Discussion with a microbiologist regarding antibiotic use is very important after getting a positive culture, and sensitivity is very important. The duration of illness varies from 7 to 14 days with the introduction of antibiotics, as advised by the microbiologist.

Case 49

1. b US of hips
   a X-ray of hips and knees
   e Urine for VMA
2. c Reduced bone density on the left
   d Fragmentation of femoral head on the left
3. a Perthes' disease

Acute painful hips

Trauma is one of the commonest causes and a detailed history will confirm this condition. In infants non-accidental injury should also be suspected if no cause can be found.

In the majority of cases, irritated hips are usually proceeded by a UTI that occurred in the previous 2–3 weeks. Affected toddlers will refuse to walk and older children will limp and have painful hips. The examination will show hips that are difficult to abduct and extend. The affected child will keep the hip and knee joints flexed, and any attempt to extend these joints will cause a lot of pain. Blood tests will be negative and a US of the hips may show free fluids; aspiration of this fluid is not indicated when all blood tests are negative. Rest and analgesia will help, and traction is not usually needed.

Osteomyelitis and septic arthritis require joint management by both a paediatrician and an orthopaedic team. The joint is usually painful to move and the child will have a fever and look septic. Inflammatory markers will be high and are useful as follow-up tools. US is vital and provides guidance to aspirating the joint. MRI or a bone scan is diagnostic, and when there are doubts, biopsy guided by CT or US is helpful. Treatment is long term in osteomyelitis with i.v. antibiotics until the inflammatory marker has normalised and the child becomes asymptomatic; then oral treatment will continue. The usual course of antibiotics will last 6–8 weeks but will be directed by clinical response and improvement in the blood and bone picture. Septic arthritis can be treated with broad-spectrum antibiotics used to cover *Staphylococcus* infection.

Other causes of painful hip joints include Henoch–Schönlein purpura, Perthes' disease, sickle-cell bone crisis, malignancy (e.g. neuroblastoma, leukaemia or osteogenic sarcoma) osteoid osteoma, histocytosis, rheumatic fever, myositis, and fractures.

Case 50

1. g NAI
2. a Admit the child and inform the duty consultant
   e Check child protection register
   d Inform Social Services and the Child Protection Team

Non-accidental injuries

Children are becoming more and more exposed to abuse. It is important to look hard for indications of NAI in order to save more children. This diagnosis is one of the most difficult to face for doctors and staff as well as carers. There is a lot of emphasis on training doctors to diagnose, recognise and deal with such cases. Children with physical injuries may not be walking yet and may have learning difficulties, an unexplainable or changing history, or changing sites of injuries. Children with a poor social background with domestic violence should be treated with a high degree of suspicion, and a thorough history and checking is required. Involving a senior colleague from the beginning is important. Documentation should be accurate, very descriptive, detailed and have no gaps. Health professionals should describe what is seen when examining the child and try to avoid giving an opinion. They should always get someone to chaperone them on examination and write their names and who else is present on the examination form. The notes should not be left with anyone until the statement or report is finished. The situation should always be discussed with the consultant as well as the lead child protection person in the treating hospital. Attending case conferences is very good experience; they can be hostile situations but the aim is to protect the child as well as the parents. Child protection teams will ask health professionals for their opinions and if this cannot be given, the child should be referred to the child protection team leader in the treating hospital.

Case 51

A 10-year-old boy presented with a history of nightmare episodes, which started at the age of 9 years. The episodes described by his mother are as follows: he wakes up with his mouth deviated to one side, unable to speak, with saliva pouring from his mouth and his arm shaking. This reaction lasts 2–3 min and then he is alright. Sometimes he falls from his bed and when his mother arrives he is confused and talking 'gibberish'. These episodes become more frequent during the week but he never misses school. He was a FTND. His father experienced the same sort of episodes but grew out of them by the age of 13 years. There is no family history of epilepsy or sleep disorders. His general and systemic examination was normal apart from a hyperpigmented patch measuring 3 × 4 cm on his left shoulder plate. His awake EEG was reported as normal. Other test results are:

BS	4.5 mmol/l
Ca	2.36 mmol/l
Mg	0.91 mmol/l
LFT	Normal
U&Es	Normal
ECG	Normal

1. What is the diagnosis?
2. What is the single most useful test?
3. What treatment should be given?

Case 52

A boy aged 7 years was referred by his doctor with a history of diarrhoea, which lasted for the preceding 4 months. He always has dirty underwear and has been bullied at school for his smell. He opens his bowel five times a day, with a runny stool and has to rush to the toilet. Fresh blood was present on three occasions, which was associated with his passing a large amount of faeces. He has not vomited and his weight is 25 kg. There has been no previous medical problem and there is no family history of a similar illness. Both parents are from west Africa and the family eats an African diet when possible. He likes bananas and sweet corn. His abdomen is soft, with a generalised fullness. His bladder is full, even if he passes urine 2 hours before the clinic appointment. There are no peri-anal lesions and no fissures.

He is the only child in the family and there is no history of travel abroad.

He does not want to go back to school and feels that his teacher will not accept him until this problem is sorted out.

The following tests were all normal: FBC, U&E, TFT, coeliac screen, ESR, CRP. Other test results are:

MSU	White cells	15
	RBC	2
Protein	Positive	
No organism		
Stool	No evidence of virus, bacterial or protozoan infection	

1. What is the most likely diagnosis?
    a   Crohn's disease
    b   Coeliac disease
    c   Cystic fibrosis
    d   Anal fistulae
    e   Constipation with overflow
    f   Ulcerative colitis
    g   Hirschsprung's disease
    h   Toddler diarrhoea
    i   Chronic protozoan infection
2. Which other investigation/s may help the diagnosis?
    a   Upper GIT endoscopy
    b   Lower GIT endoscopy
    c   Abdominal X-ray
    d   Sweat test
    e   Barium swallow and follow through
    f   Barium enema
    g   Abdominal US
    h   Repeat fresh, warm stool culture
    i   Repeat abdominal examination
3. How can this patient be managed in three steps?
    a   Start antibiotics
    b   Start oral prednisolone
    c   Give phosphate enema
    d   Start laxative (lactulose and senna)
    e   Give advice about diet
    f   Refer to surgeon for manual evacuation
    g   Refer to surgeon for surgical treatment
    h   Refer to psychologist
    i   Reassure and give no treatment
    j   Refer for genetic counselling
    k   Repeat tests after 6 months
    l   Picolax for 2 days

Case 53

A schoolboy aged 5 years presented with painful and reduced eye movement, blurred vision in his left eye and headache. His vision has been deteriorating over the last 12 hours, he can only see bright colours and any attempt to move his left eye is accompanied by severe pain. He is not able to move his left eye at all. His right eye is less painful and he can still see with it, but not as well as before. He is a keen cricket player and likes this sport. There are no other illnesses in the family and his maternal grandmother died in her 60s after a stroke-like event. He is the second child in the family; his sister is 10 years old and healthy, as is his mother, and his father is a national Rugby player.

The optic disc of the left eye is swollen and pale, with retinal exudate, and the right is normal. There is painful eye movement on the left and he can move his right eye but it is painful when he is using the lateral rectus muscle on the right. The visual field examination reveals central scatomas and the visually evoked response is delayed.

The following tests were carried out: FBC, ESR, ANA, AAs, viral titres for adenovirus, coxsackievirus, *Mycoplasma*, and Lyme disease, and all results were normal. A cranial CT with contrast was reported as normal, followed by lumbar puncture with an opening pressure of 11 mmHg. There were no cells and the protein level is 0.66 g/l.

1. What are the two most useful tests that may help the diagnosis, and in what order would you carry these out?
   a   CSF for IgG oligoclonal antibodies
   b   Cranial MRI
   c   Cranial and spinal MRI
   d   Lumbar puncture for viral PCRs
   e   Bone marrow biopsy
   f   Evoked visual potential
   g   ERG
2. What are the most likely diagnoses, and in what order would you make these?
   a   Preseptal orbital cellulitis
   b   Retrobulbar neuritis
   c   MS
   d   Septal orbital cellulitis with abscess
   e   Ethmoiditis
   f   Retinoblastoma
   g   Neuroblastoma
   h   Optic gliomas
   i   Optic neuritis
   j   Encephalomyelitis
   k   Miller–Fisher syndrome
3. Which two are appropriate methods of treatment?
   a   I.v. methylprednisolone for 3 days
   b   Optic nerve decompression
   c   Oral prednisolone for 6 weeks
   d   Aciclovir for 3 weeks
   e   i.v. antibiotics for 1 week
   f   Sinus drainage
   g   Chemotherapy
   h   Radiotherapy
   i   Physiotherapy
   j   I.v. immunoglobulin

Case 54

A boy aged 10 years presented to his doctor with loin pain. He had had this before and it was resolved with analgesia. His GP asked him to drink a lot of fluids and he has been drinking 2.5 l/d. He has to wake up three times every night to go to the toilet. His father suffers from high blood pressure, caused by nephropathy. He is very skinny and in pain. He was given codeine phosphate, which helped a little bit. After a short period he started shouting from the toilet that he was bleeding from his penis. This stopped straightaway and he was rushed for an abdominal X-ray and admitted for further management. His test results were:

Na	155 mmol/l
K	4.2 mmol/l
Cl	101 mmol/l
Ur	7.1 mmol/l
Serum osmolality	302 mosmol/kg
Urine osmolality	110 mosmol/kg
Ca	2.50
PO_4	1.6
PTH	Normal level
Phosphaturia	Negative
Amino acid urea	Negative
BS	4.5

1. What is the diagnosis?
2. Which abnormality is visible on the abdominal X-ray?

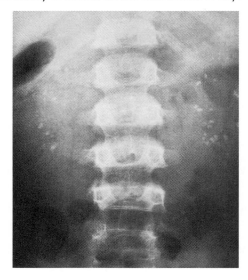

3. In which order should three other investigations be requested?

a   Urinary organic and AAs
b   Calcium/creatinine urinary clearance
c   Water deprivation test with ADDVP
d   Urine toxicology
e   Renal US
f   IVP
g   Kidney biopsy
h   24-hour urine collection for oxalate
i   Abdominal ultrasound

Case 55

A 14-year-old girl was referred by her doctor with a 2-month history of weight loss, associated with vomiting, abdominal pain and diarrhoea. She reported no blood or mucus in her stools. She also had a 1-month history of mouth ulcers, and lethargy for 1 month preceding the referral. There is no history of recent travel abroad. She has had no previous hospitalisation. There is no positive family history of ulcerative colitis in the family. She looked pale and slim, with a weight of 47.5 kg, a height of 163 cm and a BMI of 17.6. There is no evidence of finger clubbing. There is slight epigastric tenderness. There were no other abnormalities found upon systemic and general examination. The test results are:

Na	138 mmol/l
K	4.0 mmol/l
U	2.3 mmol/l
Cr	74 mmol/l
Bilirubin	6 μmol/l
ALT	8 IU/l
Alk. Ph	80 IU/l
Alb	31 g/l
Total protein	79 g/l
Ca	2.38 mmol/l
Phos	1.3 mmol/l
Mg	0.79 mmol/l
CRP	50
ESR	80 mm/hour
Hb	12.6 g/dl
WCC	6.3×10^9/l
PLT	451×10^9/l
Ferritin	5
Iron	2
γGT	118
TIBC	39
INR	1.2
Anti-endomyseal bodies	Negative
Anti-gliadin bodies	Negative
Anti-reticulin type 1	Weakly positive
Mantoux test	Negative

Igs	Normal
Stool	Negative for bacteria, parasites and viruses
ANA	Negative

1. What is the next test that should be carried out?
    a   Abdominal US
    b   Abdominal CT
    c   Abdominal MRI
    d   Upper GIT endoscopy with biopsy
    e   Lower GIT endoscopy with biopsy
    f   Barium swallow and follow through
    g   Repeat stool cultures
2. List two abnormalities that appear on her barium swallow and follow-through X-ray?

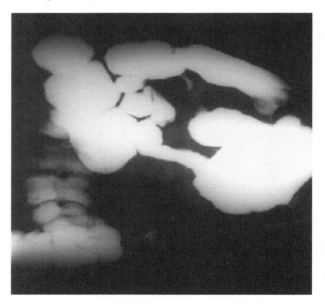

3. In what order should management steps be carried out immediately?
    a   Oral prednisolone of 2 mg/kg for 2–3 weeks
    b   Polymeric diet
    c   Azathioprine
    d   Mesalazine
    e   Metronidazole for 1 week
    f   Gluten-free diet
    g   Laparoscopy
    h   Surgical removal of affected intestine
    i   Refer to psychologist
    j   Investigate other members of family

Case 56

A 3-year-old girl presented with red eyes, which had been red on and off for the last 3 months. She now says that light hurts her eyes. She was admitted previously on two occasions with dehydration following an episode of vomiting without diarrhoea. During previous admission she was mildly acidotic, but with i.v. fluids given overnight, the situation corrected itself. She was also treated for UTI. The multisticks text shows a WCC of >100 and RBC was positive, but the test for C/S was negative. Her height and weight are on the 10th centile, and she has coarse facial features and thin hair. She is not as active as she used to be and she prefers to sit next to a radiator all of the time in winter. Her older sister is well. Both parents are from Bangladesh and are distant cousins. Her eyes look red, with no evidence of cataract or corneal opacity. The fundi examination is normal, and another systemic and general examination reveals no abnormalities apart from rough skin on her hands and legs.

Na	136 mmol/l
K	3.5 mmol/l
Ur	5.0 mmol/l
Cr	70 mmol/l
ALT	12 IU/l
Alk. Ph	150 IU/l
Bilirubin	10 μmol/l
Ca	2.30 mmol/l
Mg	0.78 mmol/l
Phosphate	1.3 mmol/l
CRP	< 5
ESR	< 2 mm/hour
TSH	30.6 mU/l
T_4	10 mU/l
Hb	12.5 g/dl
WCC	6.0×10^9/l
PLT	250×10^9/l
FSH	30 mU/l
Urine	
WCC	100
RBC	30
Cast	Red cast
Nitrite	Negative
Protein	+++
AA	Positive
pH	5.3

1. Which three non-haematological tests will help the diagnosis?
    a   Slit lamp eye examination
    b   Renal US
    c   i.v. ureterography
    d   Measuring intraocular pressure
    e   Cranial MRI

  f DMSA scan
  g Urinary GAG
  h Urinary organic acids and AAs
  i Urine for reducing substances
2. What is the most likely diagnosis?
  a Hypothyroidism
  b Lowe syndrome
  c Renal vein thrombosis
  d Lead poisoning
  e Nephrotic syndrome
  f Galactosaemia
  g Cystinosis
  h Tyrosinaemia
  i Wilson's disease
3. Which other two tests may help the diagnosis?
  a Radionuclide scan for thyroid gland
  b Urinary organic acid
  c Serum AAs
  d White cell enzyme
  e Serum lead level
  f Bone marrow aspirate
  g Serum copper and caeruloplasmin
  h Fibroblast cell culture

Case 57

A child presented with a history of pallor, headache, blurred vision and sweating. His parents mentioned that his heart races from time to time, specifically when he sweats. He feels tired and has a problem getting to sleep. His mother said that he was dribbling for 2 days, 1 month ago. His is now 7 years old and said that he has a headache that is generalised and lasts all day, but never wakes him at night or is worse during the morning. At school, there are some occasions when he needs to leave the classroom for a rest. His blood pressure is 130/80 mmHg, HR is 90 b.p.m., RR 20/min and temperature is 37.2°C. He has two hyperpigmented patches measuring 4 mm each on his torso but has no other skin lesions. There is no organomegaly and no heart murmur. All pulses are intact and his visual field and acuity are compatible with his age. The fundi are difficult to visualise as he complains that the light is hurting his eyes. His father works as a postman and his mother is a housewife. He is the youngest of three children; the older two are healthy. His grandfather died from ischaemic heart disease. The test results are:

Na	134 mmol/l
K	4.2 mmol/l
U	2.3 mmol/l
Cr	45 mmol/l
MSU	Negative
KUB US	Normal

ECHO   Normal
DMSA   Normal
Renal Doppler   Normal
Midnight cortisol < 200 mU/l
Ca   2.48 mmol/l

1. What are the three most likely differential diagnoses, and in what order would you make them?
   a   Neurofibromatosis type 1
   b   Neuroblastoma
   c   Conn's disease
   d   Chronic renal failure
   e   Phaeochromocytoma
   f   Pituitary adenoma
   g   Congenital adrenal hyperplasia
   h   Raised intracranial pressure
   i   Essential hypertension
   j   Renal artery stenosis
2. What are the most useful investigations?

Case 58

A 7-year-old girl was referred to a specialist centre with ataxia and seizures. She was an FTND and had no neonatal problems. At the age of 10 months she was seen by her GP, who diagnosed developmental delay with hypotonia. She was referred to an eye doctor for her squint, and ocular motor apraxia was diagnosed. There is strong family history of ptosis (mother and maternal grandmother). At the age of 6 years she developed absence seizures, and treatment with sodium valproate was started. An EEG performed at this stage shows spikes and waves to one side and was described as abnormal. By the age of 7 years she started to have a different type of seizure, which caused a dystonic posture of her arms that lasted for up to 20 min, her eyes rolled up and she was not able to communicate.

Two months later her ability to walk started to deteriorate, she was not able to feed herself, and myoclonic seizures emerged, associated with swinging of her head.

She is developmentally delayed, and first walked and spoke at the age of 5 years. Her memory is described by her mother as 'good', and her hearing and vision are normal.

She looks well, with a convergent squint on the left eye and a normal right eye (this was corrected at the age of 5 years). She has marked tremor, with bradykinesia and a wide base gait. Her tone is reduced, with generalised hyperreflexia. Her weight and height are on the 3rd centile and her OFC is on the 10th centile. There is an abdominal mass on the left side, not crossing the midline. The test results are:

Urea   9.1 mmol/l
Cr   87 mmol/l

Na	141 mmol/l
K	4.1 mmol/l
Ca	2.61 mmol/l
PO$_4$	1.01 mmol/l
WCC	6.1 × 10^9/l
Hb	13.2 g/dl
PLT	231 × 10^9/l
ESR	40 mm/hour
CRP	6
Abdominal US	bilateral multiple cysts affecting kidneys
Cranial MRI	Left hemispheric dysplasia, left cerebellar dysplasia, left inferior vermis absent with evidence of gliosis. Normal right hemisphere
ERG, EVP	Normal

1. Name three differential diagnoses
   a   Aicardi syndrome
   b   Joubert syndrome
   c   Idiopathic cerebral dysplasia
   d   Familial cerebral dysplasia
   e   Intoxication
   f   Spinal dysraphism
   g   Myotonic dystrophy
   h   Ataxia telangiectasia
2. Which three investigations should be performed?
   a   Alpha-fetoprotein
   b   Chromosomal study
   c   Vitamin B$_{12}$ level
   d   Biotin level
   e   EMG
   f   Immunoglobulin level
   g   CXR
   h   Slit lamp eye examination
   i   DNA linkage study

Case 59

The presence of tremor, developmental delay and hypotonia is the reason why a 5-year-old boy was referred to the outpatient department for a second opinion. He was an FTND, and had mild jaundice at birth. At the age of 5 weeks he was admitted with a history of irritability and crying; no reason for this was found. By the age of 9 weeks, during routine assessment, he was described as 'floppy' and referred for further opinion and possible investigation. He was found to be developmentally delayed, and bilateral optic atrophy was diagnosed. A full metabolic and neurophysiological investigation was carried out; no abnormality was detected. An ophthalmologist confirmed the optic atrophy, and pigmentery retinopathy was detected at this stage. At the age of 7 months he had a febrile illness associated with extrapyramidal signs and dystonia, and was described as having a 'mask face' appearance during this illness.

He had other problems: he suffered from eczema at the age of 6 months and became wheezy by the age of 8 months. Gastro-oesophageal reflux was corrected by fundoplication at the age of 1 year. He smiled at 6 weeks of age. At 18 months he was able to feed himself with his fingers. At 3 years of age he sat without support and was able to perform three-word sentences. Now at 5 years of age, he can perform five-word sentences. His vision has been described by his parents as 'able to see and look at lights'. His hearing has been tested and is normal.

There has been no such illness in the family and the parents do not want other children, as they are waiting for the opinion of a geneticist. The parents are not related. The boy has a mild, convergent squint, there are no dysmorphic features, and tremor is present. There is no dystonia, but there is generalised hypotonia with areflexia and weakness. His OFC is on the 25th centile, and his weight and height are on the 50th and 25th centile, respectively. The test results are:

Serum AA, urine organic acid and AA	Normal
MRI	High signal in white matter, not significant
EEG	Fast activity with polyspike and slow background activity
ERG	Abnormal
NCS, EMG	Normal

1. What are the three most likely diagnoses?
2. Which three other investigations should be undertaken?
3. What advice should be given to the parents?

Case 60

A 10-year-old girl presented with a history of severe scoliosis, and small and short wasted lower limbs. There is weakness on the right upper limb, with left subtle facial weakness. She attends a mainstream school. There is no bowel problem, but she wets herself during the night if she has been stressed or ill, but she was dry by day at the age of 2 years and by night by the age of 5 years. The weakness in her leg was noticed when she was 3 months of age and has been investigated. Spinal dysraphism was diagnosed and no further investigation has been carried out. Now she presents with a weakness in the right upper limb, severe scoliosis, asymmetry of the upper limbs, clumsiness with her right hand, and subtle right facial weakness with marked lower limb wasting.

She has a full range of eye movement and the results of the fundi examination are normal. The power in her upper limbs is good and she can walk downstairs while holding onto the railing. Her tone is normal, as are the reflexes in her upper limbs. Power is zero, the tone is hypotonic and reflexes are absent in the lower limbs. Sensation is intact in the upper limbs. The tactile sensation is absent in the lower limbs.

A nerve conduction study was carried out on the lower limbs and the results are as follows: the sensory part is normal and the motor part is abnormal up to T3 level. There are no abnormalities in the upper limbs, with normal overall EMG.

1. What are three possible diagnoses?
2. What diagnosis is visible on the spinal MRI?

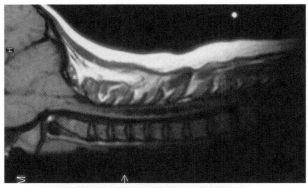

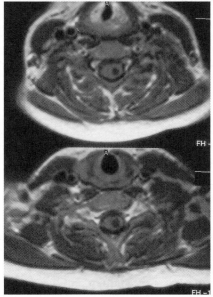

3. What other two tests should be done?

ANSWERS 51–60

Case 51

1. BRECH (benign Rolandic epilepsy of childhood)
2. Sleep EEG
3. None

Benign childhood epilepsy with centro-temporal spikes

This is a common syndrome of idiopathic partial epilepsy in childhood; the onset is between the ages of 2 and 13 years, with a mean of 7 years. It occurs in about 15–25% of school-aged children with epilepsy. It is genetically determined and it can be AS or AD. The typical seizure occurs during the night but sometimes may occur during the daytime. Sometimes children will describe a funny feeling in their mouth, which is followed by a generalised tonic–clonic seizure. These are simple partial seizures without impairment of consciousness; the warning signs are mainly motor but can be buccal or labial paraesthesia. They mainly involve the face, with salivation and/or speech arrest. Each seizure usually lasts up to 60 s. Secondary generalised seizures occur in 20% of patients with this epilepsy syndrome. The EEG is very characteristic, with centro-temporal spikes and waves during sleep recording, and quite often the awake EEG is reported as normal. No neuroimaging is required, as it will be normal. Treatment can be given to patients who are having seizures frequently, on a daily basis, and when there is parental anxiety or the school and social life of the child are affected. Seizures should respond to medication, and there is no need to give a high dose or multi-drug treatment. Carbamazepine should be avoided, as it may lead to CSS during sleep and affect school performance. The prognosis in these patients is excellent and school performance and development should not be affected. In some cases these episodes may evolve into another type of epilepsy in adult life, in the form of generalised tonic–clonic seizures.

Case 52

1. e   Constipation with overflow
2. i   Repeat abdominal examination
3. l   Picolax for 2 days
   d   Start laxative (lactulose and senna)
   e   Give advice about diet

Constipation with overflow

This is one of the commonest causes of abdominal pain. It can start at any time and usually one member of the family has had it. The cause is unknown but possible causes should be ruled out, including hypothyroidism, anal stricture, and Hirschsprung's disease. A detailed history and examination will be very helpful. There is no need to carry out an abdominal X-ray to diagnose constipation; the clinical diagnosis can be made from history and examination. Examination of the perineal region is necessary to rule out fissures or other abnormalities. A rectal examination should not be undertaken unless the history indicates the need for it. Treatment involves prescribing a stool softener and starting with a simple stimulant such as senna and lactulose. In children who are soiling their clothes, an aggressive approach with a stronger laxative is probably needed to clean them up in the first instance, then a softener and stimulant should be added. Difficult cases may need frequent enemas, which are not tolerated very well by some children. Children with a heart condition should not be prescribed strong laxatives. Involvement with a psychologist and nurse specialist is needed in difficult cases.

Case 53

1. b Cranial MRI
   a CSF for oligoclonal bands
2. i Optic neuritis
   b Retrobulbar neuritis
   d Septal orbital cellulitis with abscess
3. a i.v. methylprednisolone for 3 days
   c Oral prednisolone 2 mg/kg for 6 weeks

Optic neuritis

This is involvement of the optic nerve by inflammation, degeneration or demyelination, resulting in impaired vision and pain around the involved eye/s. Both MS and optic neuritis have the same aetiology. Some children with optic neuritis may develop MS later in life. Some viral infections may cause optic neuritis, including measles, varicella, and mumps. It can be associated with Miller Fischer syndrome. It is characterised by a sudden reduction in visual activity, either unilaterally or bilaterally. It is usually preceded by headache and painful eye movement. It usually starts by causing blurred vision and progresses to a complete loss of vision within a few days. Bilateral involvement has been reported in 75% of cases. A swollen disc can be seen in 75% of cases (neuropapillitis) and retrobulbar neuritis in 25% in a normal fundi examination. Central scatomas will be visible in a visual field examination, with delayed visually evoked response. Other causes should be excluded, such as malingering and hysteria, and other causes of optic nerve compression such as optic gliomas, pituitary adenoma (craniopharyngioma), and an AV malformation pressing on the optic nerve. Retrobulbar abscess follows septal cellulitis. An MRI scan will show demyelination of one optic nerve or both. The risk of developing MS in unilateral optic neuritis is high and the CSF may show pleocytosis and increased intrathecal IgG production of oligoclonal antibodies. No treatment has been proven to be of value but corticosteroids have been recommended in the form of methylprednisolone for 3 days and oral prednisolone for

3 weeks, which has been very helpful. The follow-up of patients with optic neuritis is very important as there is a high risk that MS may evolve. Most patients recover normal or useful vision despite the persistence of optic atrophy, but colour vision and stereoscopic vision remain impaired.

Case 54

1. Nephrogenic diabetes insipidus
2. Bilateral renal multiple high densities shadow (nephrocalcinosis)
3. Abdominal US
   a Urinary organic and AAs
   b Calcium/creatinine urinary clearance

Nephrocalcinosis

Causes
Oxalosis is an autosomal recessive inherited inborn error of metabolism, causing excessive endogenous oxalate synthesis, and there are three patterns of clinical disease: (1) malignant infantile form with nephrocalcinosis resulting in early end-stage renal failure; (2) juvenile type with recurrent stones, renal infections and oxalate deposition, which may cause arrhythmias; (3) benign adult form with less oxalate secretion and longer survival. Type 1 oxalosis results from excessive glycolate and oxalate excretion and type 2 causes excessive oxalate and L-glyceric acid excretion with normal glycolate. Diagnosis of this condition is by demonstrating high oxalate excretion and whether high or no glycolate is found in patients with renal stones or nephrocalcinosis. The metabolic enzyme defect can be detected in leukocytes in type 2 but not in type 1. Treatment is difficult, with fewer intakes of oxalate and calcium. Pyridoxine will reduce oxalate excretion in type 1, and magnesium and phosphate should be given to inhibit calcium oxalate crystal formation in the urine.

Another cause, hypercalciuria, is usually idiopathic and asymptomatic. It is sometimes present with haematuria or renal calculi and colic. The plasma calcium level is usually normal, as are levels of phosphate and parathyroid hormone. Increased gut absorption of calcium or increased bone consumption of calcium or a renal tubular defect of calcium reabsorption were suggested as causes but none could be proved. Avoiding an excessive intake of calcium and oxalate is the treatment in these cases.

Other causes include distal renal tubular acidosis, excessive vitamin D intake, sarcoidosis, renal tubular necrosis, hyperparathyroidism, hypothyroidism, prolonged immobilisation, and medullary sponge kidney.

Case 55

1. d, e, Upper and lower GIT endoscopy with biopsy
2. Cobblestone appearance, and string sign

Caseating granulomata
3. a Oral prednisolone 2 mg/kg for 2–3 weeks
    d Mesalazine
    b Polymeric diet

Crohn's disease

The aetiology of this disease is unknown and its multifactorial complex aetiology and pathology make it the most difficult inflammatory bowel disease to manage. It is a T-cell-mediated chronic inflammatory disorder that may affect any part of the GIT. Non-caseating granulomata are characteristic but not always present. It is immunological in origin but there have been many suggestions of other causes, such as bacteria, viruses or allergies. The disease is also characterised by skip areas with thick intestinal walls. It is transmural with submucosal thickening and with infiltration of lymphocytes and macrophages. The granulomata are a form of aggregated transformed macrophages that may contain giant cells. The commonest presenting features are growth failure, abdominal pain, diarrhoea and weight loss. The abdominal pain is characteristic, periumbilical, colicky and relieved by defaecation. Other features may include erythema nodosum, arthritis, uveitis and stomatitis. Perianal ulcers or fistulae may also be presenting features. Anaemia, finger clubbing, with poor weight gain and short stature, are other findings on examination. Upper GIT endoscopy as well as colonoscopy are indicated to confirm the diagnosis. The histological appearance will consist of non-caseating granulomata, fissuring ulceration, focal inflammation, submucosal or transmural inflammation, mucus retention and aggregation of lymphocytes. Barium swallow and follow-up should be performed after biopsy, but a barium enema is not needed. ESR and CRP are usually high and a way to assess patients during follow-up. Radiology can show a cobblestone appearance, aphthoid ulceration, granularity and mucosal oedema. 5-Aminosalicylic acid derivatives, elemental nutrition and surgery are the main ways of treating Crohn's disease. Steroids are used to induce remission and azathioprine can be used for its steroid-sparing effect. The prognosis is much better in paediatric patients and the risk of cancer is ill defined.

Case 56

1. h Urinary organic acid and AAs
    a Slit lamp eye examination
    b Renal US
2. g Cystinosis
3. c Serum AAs
    h Fibroblast cell culture

Cystinosis

This is a metabolic disorder that is inherited as an autosomal recessive condition; the gene is located on chromosome 17p. Prenatal diagnosis can be offered in families who have a child with cystinosis, by measuring the level of cysteine in the fibroblasts. Cysteine is usually stored intracellularly in lysosomes. The most severe form of cystinosis is the infantile type, which affects the kidneys and eyes, bone marrow and other tissues. The adult form occurs in the second decade of life, is less benign and the kidneys are usually not involved. The infantile form is characterised by a normal baby at birth, with symptoms that start to appear from the age of 6 months, including polyuria, polydipsia, FTT, dehydration, and unexplained fever with rickets. End-stage renal failure will occur within the first 10 years of life if the patient is not treated. Crystals of cysteine can be seen in the kidneys and corneas, and the cysteine level in leukocytes will be high. Fanconi syndrome due to generalised failure of proximal tubular absorption is associated with cystinosis. Careful balancing of electrolytes and nutrition is very important, as these patients are very difficult to manage. Cystemine will help to mobilize cysteine from lysosomes but, compliance is poor. Renal transplantation is effective in patients with end-stage renal failure. There is no recurrence of cystinosis in transplanted kidneys and renal function is satisfactory. Other complications associated with cystinosis include diabetes mellitus, cerebral atrophy, corneal degeneration and hypercholesterolaemia, which will arise later in life.

Case 57

1. e   Phaeochromocytoma
   b   Neuroblastoma
   a   Neurofibromatosis type1
2. Cranial MRI
   Abdominal MRI or CT
   Urinary VMA
   Urinary dopamine

Phaeochromocytoma

This is an adrenal medullary tumour that occurs more frequently than neuroblastoma and ganglioneuroma, which are very rare. It is one of the main causes of hypertension in children and occurs bilaterally in 10% of affected individuals; half of these tumours are extra-adrenal but occur in the abdomen. It is also associated with Von Hippel–Lindau syndrome and neurofibromatosis type 1. Hypertension, sweating, headache, and visual blurring are common manifestations of phaeochromocytoma. High urine levels of catecholamines their metabolites are diagnostic markers. Suppression or stimulation tests are required for the diagnostic procedure. Abdominal CT or MRI scans are needed to localise the tumour. Whole-body MIBG is required to rule out thoracic or extra-abdominal disease. Stabilising children before removing or carrying out a biopsy of the tumour is essential. An alpha-blocker drug such as oxybenzamine, and a beta-blocker such as propranolol are introduced to control tachycardia and cardiac dysarrhythmias. Fluid management is important before removing the tumour. The operation for phaeochromocytoma should be carefully planned, and invasive monitoring of BP and HR during the operation is very important. The outcome of surgery is usually good.

Case 58

1. b   Joubert syndrome
    g   Myotonic dystrophy
    h   Ataxia telangiectasia
2. a   Alpha-fetoprotein
    e   EMG
    f   Immunoglobulin level

Joubert syndrome

This syndrome consists of familial agenesis of the cerebellar vermis, episodic hyperpnoea, abnormal eye movement, ataxia and retardation. Other features include facial asymmetry, retinal anomalies, disc coloboma and renal abnormalities. The commonest presentation will be with respiratory problems, which include panting respiration interspersed with long pauses that are not associated with any changes in blood gases. Respiratory problems usually start during the neonatal period, with cyanosis. The vermis is dysplastic and cerebellar peduncles are small. The electroretinogram is flat or markedly depressed. Ataxia and retardation develop later. This syndrome can be inherited recessively but sporadic cases occur. The MRI and cranial CT will show the abnormalities. The CT appearance will show a brainstem that looks like a molar tooth. The MRI scan is more definitive and will show an umbrella-shaped sign of the lower fourth ventricle and atrophic vermis with a horizontal superior cerebellar peduncle. There are other syndromes associated with vermal agenesis, such as Dandy–Walker syndrome, Aicardi syndrome, Smith–Lemli–Opitz syndrome, Goldenhar syndrome and Meckel–Gruber syndrome.

Case 59

1. Mitochondrial disorders (recessive)
    Carbohydrate-deficient glycoprotein (CDG) syndrome
    Non-metabolic genetic disorder (Batten disease)
2. Rectal biopsy
    White cell enzymes
    Transferrin level
3. No further pregnancy until they have genetic counselling

Batten disease

This disease is characterised by storage of ceroid-lipofuscinoses lipopigments (ceroid) in the brain, which is different from pigment stored in a normal brain (lipofuscin). The lipofuscin normally accumulates over the years in a normal brain and is regarded as a normal phenomenon. Late infantile neuronal ceroid lipofuscinosis is linked to chromosome 11. Affected individuals usually present with developmental delay followed by epilepsy, usually around 30 months of age. Seizures are usually myoclonic, with erratic myoclonus. Dementia will follow; affected children will be bedridden by the age of 3–6 years and die before 10 years of age. Visual failure usually occurs late with macular, retinal degeneration and optic atrophy. The EEG is characteristic with polyspikes and a slow background rhythm, with production of spikes in the posterior region of the scalp in response to photic stimulation. The ERG is extinguished, and VEPs and somatosensory-evoked responses are very large. Suction rectal biopsy will show curvilinear inclusions, and these can be seen in vascular and smooth muscle cells, glands from skin and on a brain biopsy.

Case 60

1. Syringomyelia (syrnix)
   Spinal dysraphism
   Denervation
2. Syringomyelia (syrinx)
3. MRI of spine and brain
   Nerve conduction study to be repeated, including the pelvic floor and upper limbs

Syringomyelia

This is characterised by cavitation in the spinal cord. The cavity varies in length and may extend to the brainstem (syringobulbia). The cavity is located in the grey matter, most commonly in the cervicothoracic region. It may follow trauma or infarction. In children it is usually a congenital malformation or a cystic astrocytoma. The symptoms depend on the cyst's location. If the cyst is close to the centre of the spinal cord, pain and temperature sensations are usually affected first. Symptoms may be unilateral and sometimes involve the fingers before the shoulders when the cyst is cervical. The touch and pressure sensations will be preserved until the cyst enlarges and disturbs the posterior columns or dorsal root ganglia. A loss of pain sensation in the hands will lead to ulceration, infection and injury. Scoliosis is common and torticollis may be the initial sign in children. A large cavity may produce lower motor neurone signs in the four limbs. Sphincter control may sometimes be affected. The symptoms progress very slowly and a detailed history and examination in children presenting with paraesthesia, clumsiness, or weakness of the limbs is vital. Bulbar signs are very rare. A spinal MRI scan is diagnostic and can differentiate between astrocytoma and syringomyelia. A syringoperitoneal shunt provides the best results to decompress the cavity and prevent further deterioration.

Case 61

A girl with a known history of chronic renal failure has been on haemodialysis three times per week for the past 18 months and is waiting for a kidney transplant. Her original problem followed meningococcal septicaemia. She also needed to have her left foot amputated at that time. She is suffering from right hip pain, lethargy and muscle weakness. She is 12 years old. She says that all her bones ache, and she finds it very difficult to go upstairs and spends all her time in her bedroom on the first floor. She cannot do exercise or walk a long distance. The hip pain was associated with difficulty in flexing her hips. Her BP is stable and her BM is 4.5 mmol/l. Her hip US was reported as normal and an X-ray of the long bones shows osteopenia and reduced mineralisation.

1. What abnormality is visible on this X-ray?

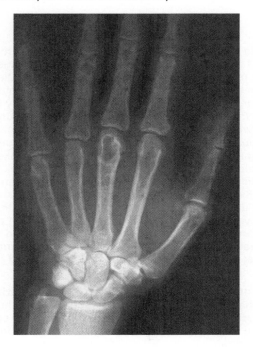

2. What are the two causes of these bone abnormalities?
    a   Rickets
    b   Secondary hyperparathyroidism
    c   Chronic renal failure
    d   Metabolic acidosis

    e   Aluminium toxicity
    f   Renal dialysis
    g   1,25(OH)$_2$D$_3$ deficiency
    h   Infection
    i   Reactive arthritis
    j   Malignancy
    k   JCA
3. What is the diagnosis?
    a   Chronic renal failure
    b   Renal osteodystrophy, secondary to chronic renal failure
    c   Hyperparathyroidism
    d   Distal renal tubular acidosis
    e   Fanconi syndrome
    f   Familial hypophosphataemic rickets
    g   JCA
    h   Psoriatic arthritis
    i   SLE

Case 62

A 2-year-old girl was born at term with no neonatal problems until the age of 1 month, when she was seen by a GP because she was floppy, not moving her legs and not interested in feeding. She was admitted to the local hospital and treated with antibiotics for 2 days, then discharged home on day 4, with the diagnosis by US of GOR. Anti-reflux medication was started and she was well until the age of 5 months, when this started to happen again. She became floppy, could not bear weight on her feet and lost her head control. She was also having a problem with feeding as she would choke on her food. These episodes of floppiness happen once every week. The anti-reflux medication was stopped and she was only given Gaviscon. At the age of 6 months all medication was stopped and she seemed to be all right until the age of 11 months. When she started crawling, her legs were weak and gave way. She was not able to sit properly. An EEG was carried out during one of these episodes and was reported to be normal. She was referred to a specialised unit and a full metabolic screen, including a fasting test, was carried out. All results came back normal.

At the age of 18 months she started to fall over, and with these episodes she was blinking her eyes quite frequently throughout. An EEG was carried out ictally and post-ictally, and was reported to be normal. The result of an ophthalmological examination of VEP and ERG was normal. A brain MRI was found to be normal. Now these episodes happen three to four times per week. They last up to 5 min each time and following these her gait is affected. Some of these episodes can last up to 1 hours. Recently she started yawning, blinking her eyes quite often and turning her head to one side during these attacks. Following an attack she feels tired and goes to sleep for up to 1 hour. She had five UTIs investigated fully and no abnormalities were found. She is the only child of healthy middle-class parents, who both work from home. There is no such illness or history of headaches or epilepsy in the family. Upon a general or systemic examination, no abnormalities were found. The results of a central nervous system (CNS) examination were normal but her mother insists that her gait is not as it should be. The girl was admitted for video telemetry for 2 days. She had three attacks, which have been described as follows: she goes pale, her eyes move horizontally and she lies motionless during each attack, which lasts between 30 and 60 s. There is no evidence of abnormality on the EEG that is associated with these attacks.

1. What is the most likely diagnosis?
   a Vasovagal attacks
   b Seizures
   c Vertigo
   d Benign paroxysmal vertigo
   e Ataxia
   f Dystonia
   g Migraine
   h Transient ischaemic attack
   i Dancing eye syndrome
2. What is the appropriate treatment?

Case 63

A 4-year-old child presented with weight and height < 3rd centile. He is not eating and his BMI is 17. He vomits at least four times/week, is lethargic and complains of abdominal pain that is not located centrally. He passes between 0.5 and 1 L of urine each day. He also drinks a lot but does not eat much. His father died from a bowel disease 1 year ago. He suffers from cramps in his legs and for some time he was unable to walk (as if he is paralysed). He has two older sisters, who are healthy and doing well at school. He looks very thin but is still active and cheerful. He has no skin marks or organomegaly. His blood pressure is 80/60 mmHg, his fundi are normal, as is the result of a CNS examination. His CXR is described as normal, but his abdominal US is abnormal, with multiple echogenic masses in his kidneys, although his liver and spleen are normal. Other test results are:

Na	138 mmol/l
K	2.3 mmol/l
U	4.2 mmol/l
Cr	60 mmol/l
Cl	102 mmol/l
HCO_3	14 mmol/l
Ca	2.12 mmol/l
pH	1.35 mmol/l
BM	4.5 mmol/l
Osmolality	297 mosmol/l

MSU

pH	6.1
WCC	10
BCs	5
Calcium/creatinine ratio	High
Osmolality	200 mosmol/l

1. What are the most likely causes?
    a   Fanconi syndrome
    b   Chronic renal failure
    c   Nephrogenic diabetes insipidus
    d   Distal renal tubular acidosis (TA)
    e   Proximal renal TA
    f   Hypercalciuria
    g   Primary hyperparathyroidism
    h   Primary hypothyroidism
2. What is the diagnosis?
3. Which four other investigations may help the diagnosis?
    a   Ammonium chloride loading test
    b   Serum AAs
    c   Water deprivation test
    d   PTH
    e   TSH/T$_4$
    f   Calcium/Cr ratio
    g   Chromosomes
    h   IVU
    i   DMSA scan
    j   Urine organic acid and AAs

Case 64

A toddler presented with her mother and had a history of having been unwell for the past 7 days. This started with a high temperature. She wouldn't eat and was irritable. This lasted for 2 days, then she developed a rash all over her body, which started at her neck and then spread. The GP saw her at this time and diagnosed a viral rash. Her temperature stayed down for another 5 days but then she had a very high temperature again, with rigors and irritability. Her mother gave her paracetamol overnight, but the girl was still not able to sleep and was described by her mother as 'jumpy all night'. She is one of seven children, of a travelling family that now lives in a caravan. Three of her elder sisters and one brother have been unwell before her, with a similar illness and rash, but recovered within 5 days and only have the remains of the rashes on their bodies. The mother also said that all of them had watery eyes and were drooling. There is no peeling of the skin and there are no joint problems. The toddler is 18 months old and her mother is not sure which of her children have been vaccinated and which have not, but she thinks her daughter has had the vaccine (BPT + polio and Hib) only once. There are a dog and a cat living with the family. The parents want to move the family to another site as soon as their daughter starts to get better. The girl is febrile and miserable, has a fading rash, and a RR 45/min, a HR of 140 b.p.m., Sat level of 89% in air and 95% on 4 L O_2 via a facemask. There is marked intercostal recession, with coarse crepitation on both lungs. The liver is 1 cm enlarged and there is no splenomegaly. There is no heart murmur and she is alert. She was admitted and had a CXR, which was described as showing bronchopneumonia (pneumonitis) with multiple small lesions in both lungs below the right costal margin. The test results are:

CRP	250
Hb	9.4 g/dl
WCC	24×10^9/l (N 40%, L 58%)
PLT	350×10^9/l
ESR	10
Ig	Normal
CD4/CD8 ratio	Normal
CH50	Normal
Heaf test	No reaction
Sweat test	Na < 40 mmol/l

1. What other investigation/s may help the diagnosis?
   a   Bronchoscopy with lavage
   b   Chest CT
   c   Measles IgM antibodies
   d   Rubella IgM antibodies
   e   NPA
   f   Echocardiography
   g   Mantoux test 1:1000
   h   HIV antibody
   i   *Mycoplasma* titres
   j   Gastric wash for *Mycobacterium*
2. What is the most likely diagnosis from the CXR?
   a   HIV infection
   b   Giant-cell pneumonitis
   c   Cystic fibrosis
   d   Diamond–Schwachman syndrome
   e   Combined immune deficiency syndrome
   f   Foreign body
   g   Bronchiectasis
   h   Interstitial pneumonia

Case 65

A 7-year-old boy was found in his bed, having a generalised tonic–clonic seizure early one morning. He presented twice to A & E with an altered level of consciousness following a UTI. The night before, he had been unwell. The next morning, he vomited, was drowsy and suddenly started fitting. A BM test showed a glucose level of 1.1 mmol/l, which was confirmed by laboratory result. A urine test shows +++ ketones, ++ proteins and no organisms. He complains of muscle pains. He had had another admission from the outpatient department, with a blood glucose level of 2.2 mmol/l in the past. A PMH and FH test showed left VUR, which was diagnosed when he was 5 months old. He had had two other admissions in Seoul, South Korea, for similar episodes, and also had had a febrile convulsion when he was 3 years old.

Plasma AA, lactate, NH_4, very-long-chain fatty acids, GH, cortisol, and TFT levels were all within normal values. Urine organic acid and AAs were normal.

1. What is the most likely cause of his seizures?
   - a   Lack of sleep
   - b   Hypoglycaemia
   - c   High ketones in urine
   - d   High blood pressure
   - e   Uraemia
2. What is the most likely diagnosis?
3. How could the diagnosis be confirmed?

Case 66

At the age of 11 years, a young girl presented to A&E with joint pain and was not feeling well. She was treated for an episode of tonsillitis 6 weeks ago, which she recovered from completely but has felt tired ever since then. She has a rash on her back and lower limbs that looks like bruises. She finds it very difficult to sleep without using three pillows under her head, as her breathing is much better with these. Her father died from a brain tumour 3 years ago. Both her sister and brother are well. Her mother is a full-time teacher, and two cats and three goldfish live in the house with them. She does not go to school any more as she is too tired. Upon expiration, a gallop rhythm with early diastolic murmur at the mid-sternal edge can be heard. A soft systolic murmur can also be heard at the apex. An ejection systolic click can be heard at the lower sternal edge. The liver measures 3 cm below the costal margin, and has a smooth surface. The test results are:

Na	141 mmol/l
K	3.9 mmol/l
U	6.2 mmol/l
Cr	55 mmol/l
Ca	2.12 mmol/l
Alb	36 g/l
Total protein	70 g/l
ALT	35 IU/l
Alk. Ph	280 IU/l
Hb	11.2g/dl
WCC	6.9×10^9/l
PLT	450×10^9/l
INR	1.1
PTT	50 s

ANA	Negative
ReF	Negative
ESR	50 mm/hour
CRP	25

1. What are the most urgent investigations?
    a   ECG
    b   MRI of heart
    c   Catheterisation
    d   Echocardiography
    e   CXR
    f   Abdominal US
    g   X-ray of knees
    h   24-hour ECG
2. Which three other investigations are appropriate?
    a   ASO titres
    b   Throat swab
    c   Anti-DNase
    d   Blood film
    e   Blood culture
    f   DNA double strand
    g   CK
    h   Chromosomes
    i   AAs
    j   Sweat test
    k   Ig
    l   Thyroid function
    m   Viral titres for: coxsackievirus, adenovirus, parvovirus and
        EBV

An ECHO was performed and showed that the anterior mitral valve
leaflet was thickened and the posterior leaflet was moving
paradoxically. There is mild mitral regurgitation. The aortic valve is
bicuspid with AR flow velocity. The AR flow velocity was 3 m/s with a
gradient of 36 mm. The peak systolic flow across the valve was 2 m/s.

3. What lesions are associated with ECHO and clinical findings?
    a   Mitral valve stenosis
    b   Aortic stenosis
    c   Bicuspid aortic valve stenosis
    d   Mitral valve prolapse
    e   Mitral regurgitation
    f   ASD
    g   VSD
    h   Pulmonary stenosis
    i   Tricuspid regurgitation
4. What is the diagnosis?
    a   Acute rheumatic fever
    b   Endocarditis
    c   Congenital heart disease
    d   Myocarditis

e   JCA
f   SLE

Case 67

A 13-year-old girl was admitted to hospital with a history of deterioration in her dystonic movements in the last 2 days. She is known to have dystonic cerebral palsy. Co-careldopa helped slightly and she was given 10 mg oral diazepam when needed. She had had diarrhoea, which stopped 24 hours before admission. She was born at term without pre- or postnatal problems. Her problem started at the age of 2 years, when she couldn't walk and developed abnormal movement, and since then her global development has been behind. She is conscious and able to communicate with her mother, but the dystonic movements continue and she finds it very distressing. The dose of Co-careldopa was increased to 125 mg/twice a day and she was given one dose of chloral hydrate and 10 mg of oral diazepam. She was still having violent dystonic movements 1 hour later, and the results of the blood tests are:

Na	130 mmol/l
K	4.7 mmol/l
Ur	6 mmol/l
Cr	120 mmol/l
ALT	55 IU/l
Alk. Ph	330 IU/l
Hb	14 g/dl
PLT	250×10^9/l
CRP	< 5
ESR	< 2 mm/hour
Urine	Positive for blood
Stool	Negative

1. What is the most likely diagnosis?
    a   Status epilepticus
    b   Choreoathetotic crisis
    c   Sydenham chorea
    d   Parkinsonian-like crises
    e   Oculojerk crisis
2. What are three other important tests?
    a   EEG
    b   ASO titres
    c   Daily CK
    d   Urine myoglobulin
    e   Muscle biopsy
    f   Urine toxicology
    g   Co-careldopa level
    h   Cranial MRI
    i   EMG
    j   Daily U&E's
3. List the correct steps of her management

a   Rehydration
b   Regular sedation with diazepam
c   Regular sedation with chloromethiazole
d   Maximise L-dopa
e   Ventilate and sedate
f   Daily CK and U&Es
g   Transfer to PICU
h   Regular analgesia

Case 68

A male infant was seen in the rapid access clinic with a history of tachypnoea and no feeding for the last 48 hours. He was a full-term normal vaginal delivery. His mother is a refugee from Zimbabwe and he has two older siblings, aged 4 and 6 years, who are well and healthy. The father has obtained a visa to enter Britain in the last 7 months. The boy is now 4 months old and has been totally breast-fed while they live in a refuge-detention centre. His weight is 4.600 kg, OFC is 42 cm, HR 120 b.p.m., RR 30/min, Sat level in air 91% with intercostal recession, and there is subcostal recession. Air entry is reduced in both bases, and there are no added sounds. His spleen measures 3 cm and there is one large cervical gland on the left side of his neck. He is sleepy. O_2 was given at a rate of 5 l/min via a facemask with a reservoir, and the Sat picked up to 95–97%. He has large tonsils and there are two birthmarks on his abdomen. He was admitted for investigation and treatment. His test results are:

Hb	9.6 g/dl
WCC	$15.9 \times 10^9/l$
PLT	$250 \times 10^9/l$
ALT	25 IU/l
Alk. Ph	125 IU/l
TSH	1.56 mU/l
T_4	15 mU/l
CRP	145
IgG	22.2
IgA	5.4
IgE	< 2
Abdominal US	Large spleen measuring 3 cm
MSU	Negative
Mantoux test	1:10000 & 1:1000 Negative

1.   Which two abnormalities appear on the CXR?
    a   Hyperinflation
    b   Consolidation of the lower lobes
    c   Bilateral prominent hilars
    d   Bilateral nodular infiltration
    e   Pulmonary oedema
    f   Increased bronchial wall thickening
    g   Right upper lobe opacity
    h   Interstitial granulation in both lung fields

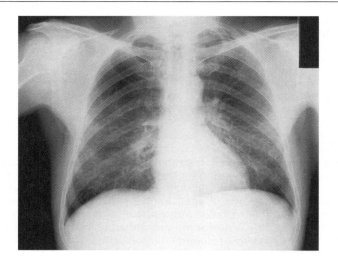

2. What is the most likely diagnosis?
    a   Bronchiolitis
    b   Aspiration pneumonia
    c   Congestive heart failure
    d   *Pseudomonas carinii* pneumonia (PCP)
    e   Pulmonary tuberculosis
    f   Cystic fibrosis
    g   Allergic alveolitis
    h   Bronchopneumonia
3. Which three other tests should be carried out?
    a   HIV antibody
    b   pH study
    c   Sweat test
    d   PG24
    e   NPA
    f   Lymph node biopsy
    g   Heaf test
    h   CD4/CD8 ratio
    i   Bone marrow biopsy
    j   Bronchial lavage for PCP
    k   Lateral CXR
    l   ECHO

Case 69

A 2½-year-old presented with a history of developmental delay, FTT, photosensitivity, scoliosis, tremor, no tears, and rashes from the age of 1 year. She was an FTND and there were no neonatal problems. Her development was normal for the first 6 months, when she had chickenpox and recovered without a problem. The OFC at the age of 8 months was below the 3rd centile. She sat at age of 14 months and she started to walk a few steps. At this time she had no language and was wearing spectacles for short-sightedness. Her hearing is normal. Tremors started at the age of 1 year and sometimes can be very bad. The tremors are mainly proximal and sometimes there is a period of up to 1 month without any tremors. The skin rash started on the upper limbs and has now disappeared. It is eczema-like rash in a lineal pattern on exposed areas. Scoliosis was noticed at the age of 1 year and has become more prominent recently. She was referred to a hospital outpatient department with a history of FTT, was diagnosed as having GOR, and is currently receiving treatment for this. Her weight, height and OFC are still below the 3rd centile. Her mother describes her as a 'dry baby' as she never noticed any tears during episodes of crying. There is no such family history, and the parents are Caucasian and not related. Examination revealed a small child with severe scoliosis, sunken eyes and a small head. She is constantly drooling. She stands with the support of a chair and can only walk one or two steps without support. She has no skin problems, all reflexes are absent in the lower limbs and reduced in upper limbs, and she has stiff legs. Tremor is marked in her hands.

A fundoscopy shows pigmentary retinopathy. Her tongue is described by a maxillofacial surgeon as 'smooth without fungiform papillae'.

The following investigations were carried out and are all normal: chromosomes, AAs, organic acids, lactate, NH_4, CSF lactate and pyruvate, brain MRI, EMG and a skin biopsy. An NCV was carried out and axonal neuropathy was suggested.

1. What are three differential diagnoses?
2. List four further investigations.
3. What three steps should form the management plan?

Case 70

A 9-year-old girl presented with a history of joint pain, fever and headache. She had lost 6 kg in the past 2 months, was increasingly lethargic and had poor concentration. Her blood pressure was measured by her GP when she was 8 years old and was 110/75 mmHg; at this time she presented with a rash all over her body that was described as 'a small pinpoint rash'. This rash disappeared after advice from a paediatrician to give a 5-day course of oral prednisolone on the basis of diagnosis of Henoch–Schönlein purpura. Her blood pressure was never checked again. A headache started 2 days ago and is severe enough for her to find it difficult even to chew. Paracetamol helped for 2 hours only. The pinpoint rash comes and goes but she never bothered to ask for help as she has been told it is benign and will go in time. Her BP was 130/80 mmHg on three occasions. The rash is mainly on her arms and legs and is present to a lesser degree on her face and chest; it does not blanch when pressed. She is afebrile at the moment but her temperature can be high on some days. The longest period she has had without a temperature was 7 days, 2 weeks ago, after a course of antibiotics and non-steroidal anti-inflammatory drugs (NSAIDs). No other abnormalities were found on systemic examination, apart from a swollen left ankle joint. An X-ray of the joint showed soft-tissue swelling. Other test results are:

LFT and U&Es	Normal
ESR	70 mm/hour
CRP	25
Ferritin	1600
PLT	345 × 10⁹/l
DNA double strand	Negative
Renal US	Normal
Cranial CT	Normal with contrast
Hb	12.5 g/dl
WCC	6.8 × 10⁹/l
ANA	Weakly positive

1. What other tests may help the diagnosis?
   a   Renal artery angiography
   b   Renal biopsy
   c   Pin-point lesion biopsy
   d   HBsAg
   e   Lyme disease serology
   f   DMSA scan
   g   Cranial diffuse weight (DW) MRI
   h   Muscle biopsy
   i   Joint biopsy
   j   *Mycoplasma* titres
   k   Skin biopsy
   l   Renal US
2. What are the most likely diagnoses in order?
   a   JCA
   b   SLE
   c   Kawasaki disease
   d   Henoch–Schönlein purpura
   e   Behçet's syndrome
   f   Lyme disease
   g   Hepatitis B
   h   Polyarteritis nodosa
   i   Phaeochromocytoma
   j   Renal TB
   k   Ehlers–Danlos syndrome
   l   Scleroderma
   m   Mixed connective-tissue disorders

ANSWERS 61–70

Case 61

1. Renal osteodystrophy
2. c Chronic renal failure
   a Rickets
3. b Renal osteodystrophy secondary to chronic renal failure

Renal osteodystrophy

This is due to disturbances in bone and mineral metabolism secondary to chronic renal failure. Phosphate retention, secondary hyperparathyroidism, skeletal resistance to parathyroid hormone, hypocalcaemia due to malabsorption of calcium, and changes to vitamin D metabolism in patients with chronic renal failure are biochemical changes associated with renal osteodystrophy. Severity is mainly related to time of onset, of renal failure and to the cause. It is worse with congenital causes. If the GFR is more than 25 ml/min/1.73m², renal dystrophy is very unlikely to occur. Many skeletal symptoms are associated with this, including poor growth (short stature), bone pain, and skeletal abnormalities. 1-Alpha-hydroxycholecalciferol should be given when biochemical changes start to appear in patients with chronic renal failure (hypocalcaemia, hyperphosphataemia, a rise in alkaline phosphatase or hyperparathyroidism) or if the GFR falls below 25 ml/min/1.73m². Dietary phosphate restriction and phosphate binders (calcium bicarbonate) are effective, and aluminium hydroxide use should be avoided in children. Renal transplantation is the best replacement therapy in patients with chronic renal failure and associated complications.

Case 62

1. d Benign paroxysmal vertigo
2. Good and no treatment is required

Benign paroxysmal vertigo

This is a disorder of infants and preschool children. It is characterised by a sudden onset of vertigo, with difficulty in maintaining posture. The child will lie motionless on the floor, or indicate the need to be held by a parent. Ataxia and headaches are not associated with these events. The child will be pale, exhibit nystagmus and be frightened. These episodes may last a minute or two. The attacks may be replaced by headache and vomiting as time passes. A family history of migraine is always present. No treatment is required, but antimigraine treatment can be given, especially if attacks are associated with headache.

Case 63

1. g Primary hyperparathyroidism
   h Primary hypothyroidism
   a Fanconi syndrome
   b Chronic renal failure
   f Hypercalciuria
2. Distal renal TA
3. a Ammonium chloride loading test
   d PTH
   e TSH/T$_4$
   b Serum AAs
   j Urine organic acid and AAs

Distal renal TA

In the classic type of distal renal TA, there is an inability to lower urinary pH below 5.8 and an inability to excrete appropriate amounts of acid, even when a loading acid dose is given. It can be diagnosed by an ammonium chloride loading dose that fails to lower urinary pH below 5.8; urinary acid excretion will be reduced. There are many causes, which can be idiopathic or familial, including deafness, or secondary to nephrocinosis, hypercalcaemia, renal parenchymal lesions, and vitamin D intoxication. It is transient in infants.

It is sporadic, and children can present with anorexia, vomiting, and FTT. Chronic acidosis may lead to chronic bone disease, as there will be excessive removal of calcium from bones to be secreted in the urine; this may also lead to renal calculi and polyuria. There will be a low level of potassium as a result of increased distal sodium. Potassium exchange can also cause polyuria. The potassium level can be very low, which may cause cardiac arrhythmias, flaccid paralysis, respiratory difficulties and coma. Sodium bicarbonate will correct acidosis completely and growth will return to normal. In nephrocalcinosis the changes will take time and may not return to normal. A potassium supplement is required in cases where there is symptomatic hypokalaemia.

Case 64

1. c Measles IgM antibodies
2. Giant cell pneumonitis

Measles

Presentation usually accompanies fever, respiratory tract symptoms, a runny nose (coryza), cough, and conjunctivitis. Koplik's spots on mucosal membranes – small (1–3 mm), irregular, bright red spots, with a bluish-white speck at centre – may be enormous in number; red areas may become confluent. A maculopapular rash extends from the face to the lower body and mainly limbs. Recovery is usually rapid, but it is important that the patient has an unimpaired cell-mediated immune response. There is continued growth in the lungs, leading to giant-cell pneumonia. Since the virus grows in the epithelia of the nasopharynx, middle ear, and lungs, all of these sites may then be susceptible to secondary bacterial infection. Otitis media and bacterial pneumonia are quite common. The outcome is affected by the state of nourishment of the patient and access to medical care. Measles is still a major killer in underdeveloped countries. Interstitial pneumonia and pneumonia accounts for 60% of deaths from measles. One in 1000 cases may get encephalitis a few days after the rash disappears. Most patients survive encephalitis but there may be complications – deafness, seizures, and mental disorders.

Subacute sclerosing panencephalitis

Very rarely (seven in 1 000 000 cases), the patient may get subacute sclerosing panencephalitis (SSPE). This develops 3–10 years after initial infection. It is a progressive, fatal disease. Affected children will present with frequent falls, myoclonic jerks – especially on touch – progressive dementia, and an encephalopathic picture. EEG is very characteristic, with paroxysmal complexes in the form of high-voltage slow waves recruiting periodically at the time of the clinical jerks. This may be seen even before the child becomes severely symptomatic. Risk factors include a history of primary measles at an early age. The incidence of SSPE has decreased since the advent of vaccination. SSPE is associated with defective forms of the virus in the brain, and so it is difficult to isolate the infectious virus from such patients. Certain viral proteins are often not expressed; the M protein is frequently absent. The CSF contains no cells and the protein level is normal. The immunoglobulins, mainly IgG, are always high, with an oligoclonal pattern. Specific antibodies for measles are present in CSF as well as blood and at very high levels, as well as in the serum. This is a fatal condition and the duration of the disease is usually less than 12 months. There is no treatment yet but supportive care for the patients and family is very important.

Measles is one of the preventable infectious diseases and has been almost abolished since the introduction of the measles vaccine in many countries. Many new cases have been reported in babies whose parents decided not to give the measles, mumps and rubella vaccine for fear of autism and inflammatory bowel diseases. No link has yet been proven between the triple vaccine (MMR) and autism and inflammatory bowel disease.

Case 65

1. b   Hypoglycaemia
2. Ketotic hypoglycaemia
3. Fasting and test blood for: ketones, glucose, acetylcarnitine, cortisol level, GH, and very-long-chain fatty acids

Ketotic hypoglycaemia

This condition occurs frequently in small, poorly growing infants and children. A lack of glycogen storage and muscle protein for gluconeogenesis will cause an increase in lipolysis. The child will use the fatty acids, and ketones will be accumulated. In these children the plasma alanine and lactate levels are low but a normal response to intramuscular (IM) glucagon challenge is shown. Children with the fatty acid oxidation defect will show progressive symptoms with lethargy, nausea, hypoglycaemia, hyperketosis, progressive somnolence and hepatic encephalopathy. Young children may have muscle weakness, hypotonia, delayed development, exercise intolerance, muscle pain and cramps. This can be diagnosed by studying the organic acids and carnitine status. Plasma acetyl-carnitine or acetylglycine profiles by fast-atom bombardment/mass spectrometry often help the diagnosis. Enzyme assays can be carried out on white cells or cultures of skin fibroblasts. Avoidance of fasting and a ready regime of non-fat calories, given orally, can be advised when needed. L-Carnitine is indicated in all fatty oxidation defects. Other causes of ketotic hypoglycaemia include glycogen storage disease, and pyruvate, citric acid cycle and organic acid metabolism.

Case 66

1. d ECHO
   a ECG
   e CXR
2. a ASO titres
   b Throat swab
   e Blood culture (three times)
3. e Mitral regurgitation
   c Bicuspid aortic valve stenosis
4. a Acute rheumatic fever

Acute rheumatic fever

This causes significant morbidity and mortality in the paediatric age group. It is relatively rare in developed countries but common in developing countries. Carditis is the commonest manifestation, which will cause permanent damage. There will be a history of throat infection or tonsillitis 2–3 weeks prior to this. Polyarthritis moves from one joint another, usually the large joints such as the knees, ankles, and elbows. Chorea, subcutaneous nodules and erythema marginatum are other major manifestations. The minor criteria include rheumatic heart disease, arthralgia, fever, a high CRP or ESR, leukocytosis, a prolonged PR interval and previous rheumatic fever. Diagnosis of acute rheumatic fever should be expected in patients with two major or one major and two minor signs. Carditis affects at least two-thirds of patients. The appearance or worsening of heart murmur, pericarditis and heart failure is an indication of carditis. The apical systolic murmur is one typical murmur that indicates mitral regurgitation. A short apical mid-diastolic murmur will indicate mitral regurgitation and, less commonly, the high-pitched decrescendo, early diastolic murmur will indicate aortic regurgitation. Pericarditis can be recognised by pericardial friction rub and is always associated with myocarditis and valvular lesions. ECG may show a prolonged PR interval, complete heart block, and flattened or inverted T-wave on V4–V6, characteristic of pericarditis. Echocardiography will help to determine the state of the myocardium and any pericardial effusions. It is important that the affected child have bed rest. Use of oral penicillin, salicylate, and corticosteroids for 10 days should only follow severe carditis or heart failure. Prophylaxis should be given to all patients with previous acute rheumatic fever. Phenoxypenicillin should be administered in a dose of 125 mg twice/day; if the patient is allergic to penicillin, sulphadiazine or erythromycin can be used. The prognosis is worse if there is aortic valve involvement or progressive cardiac dilatation.

Case 67

1. b   Choreoathetotic crisis
2. c   Daily CK
   j   Daily U&E's
   d   Urine myoglobulin
3. a   Rehydration (fluid intake should be 100 ml/kg/day, oral or i.v.)
   b   Diazepam every 6 hours and/or 2 hourly chloromethiazole
   h   Regular analgesia

Dystonia

This is a disturbance of posture caused by simultaneous contracture of agonist and antagonist muscles. The posture initiates movement in the face, limbs, and trunk. There may be focal dystonia in the face, called blepharospasms, which may be caused by drugs, encephalitis, hysteria, myotonia, seizures, hemi-facial spasms, Wilson disease, and Huntington's chorea. There is generalised dystonia, which may be caused by metabolic disorders such as cytochrome b deficiency, dopa-responsive dystonia, gluthatic aciduria, Wilson disease and many other causes. This condition also involves segmental and hemi-dystonia. Choreoathetotic crisis may follow generalised dystonia. It is usually preceded by a viral illness and will cause the child to have non-stop muscular movement, which will affect sleep. As this movement is violent and painful, the child will be tired and dehydrated. The CK will be very high and muscles will be damaged; this will lead to severe myoglobinuria, which will lead to renal failure if not recognised and treated early. Patients with these crises should be overhydrated, and given regular painkillers, and blood should be taken daily to assess renal function. Other drugs that may aid sleep and sedation include diazepam, chlormethiazole, and melatonin. Levodopa is effective in some patients, but the dose should be increased very slowly after initial administration. Looking for a cause is important for genetic counselling and prognosis. Detailed investigations including muscle and skin biopsies are worthwhile to help the parents and child.

Case 68

1. a Hyperinflation
   h Interstitial granulation in both lung fields
2. d PCP
3. h CD4/CD8 ratio
   a HIV antibody
   j Bronchial lavage for PCP

Interstitial pneumonitis (*Pneumocystis carinii* pneumonia)

Pneumocystis carinii has many features of a fungus. Immune-compromised children are most vulnerable to infection with this organism. Cystic fibrosis is another disease that will affect children in the first 4 years of life. Children with T-cell defects are more vulnerable to infection, and this can lead to PCP. The clinical features of PCP develop very slowly and consist of dyspnoea on exertion or tachypnoea at rest, a dry cough, breathlessness and cyanosis. There are few auscultatory signs found and the CXR will show diffuse infiltrates that can resemble a ground glass appearance. The blood gases will show a low oxygenation rate and low CO_2. Sputum, if found, will contain a characteristic cyst, with special staining (silver methenamine). This can also be found on the nasopharyngeal aspirate, bronchial lavage or lung biopsy. Monoclonal antibodies will help to identify *P. carinii*. A high dose of co-trimoxazole for a period of 14–21 days should be given, and if there is no response, i.v. pentamidine can be used. Steroids in HIV infection and PCP show a reduction in the mortality rate for these conditions. Children with PCP secondary to *P. carinii* should be given prophylaxis (co-trimoxazole) either daily or three times per week. Other causative factors for PCP are *Mycoplasma pneumoniae*, CMV, and *Legionella*.

Case 69

1. Riley–Day syndrome
   Rett syndrome
   Cockayne syndrome
2. Spinal and brain MRI
   Awake and sleep EEG
   ERG, EVP
   Repeat skin biopsy
3. Genetic counselling
   Refer to orthopaedic surgeon
   Review by ophthalmologist

Hereditary sensory and autonomic neuropathy type III (Riley–Day syndrome)

This syndrome is transmitted as an autosomal recessive trait and is common in Ashkenazi Jews (chromosome 9p31–q33). It is characterised by a loss of neurons in the posterior root, Lissauer tract and intermediolateral grey columns, and loss of unmyelinated and myelinated fibres in peripheral nerves where a catecholamine ending is lacking. The onset of symptoms occurs from the first few days of life with hypotonia, sucking difficulties, a poor cry and vomiting. As the child grows up, other features incude growth retardation, absence of tears, skin blotching, motor incoordination, unstable temperature and BP, cyclic vomiting, and drooling. Death in infancy and early childhood is due to apnoea and chest infection. Scoliosis, postural hypotension and impaired gastric motility are major problems associated with this condition. Absence of fungiform papillae in the tongue is one of the diagnostic criteria. Absent or diminished tendon reflexes and meiosis on instillation of 2.5% metacholine histamine in the eyes are other features in helping the diagnosis of Riley–Day syndrome. Treatment is supportive, and diazepam and chlorpromazine are effective in treating acute crises and hypertension. Prenatal diagnosis is possible and the prognosis is poor.

Case 70

1. c   Pin-point lesion biopsy
   a,   Renal artery angiography
   l   Renal US
   g   Cranial DW MRI
2. h   Polyarteritis nodosa
   m   Mixed connective-tissue disorders
   b   SLE

Polyarteritis nodosa

This is a necrotising vasculitis of small and medium-sized muscular arteries. Multiorgan involvement is associated with this condition in the form of angiographic features of aneurysms. Symptoms are varied but usually are associated with fever on and off, irritability, weight loss and lethargy. Various skin rashes arise in different stages of the disease. The arteritis involving the liver, kidneys, heart and GIT will produce symptoms and signs related to the affected organ. The pathology in small- and medium-sized muscular arteries is characterised by polymorphonuclear infiltration and necrosis. Anti-nuclear antibodies are high in the majority of patients. The ESR will be high but the diagnosis can be made by biopsy from the skin lesions, kidney, or liver. The prognosis is usually poor, with many complications such as renal failure, hypertension, strokes, hypertensive retinopathy, liver failure and GIT problems. Steroids can be helpful, and other options for immunotherapy should be considered.

Case 71

An adopted girl aged 3 years presented with a history of possible vision problems. Her mother said that in the last 2 weeks she has always looked at her books in a funny way – usually at a sharp angle to her eyes. Sometimes she puts them very close to her eyes. She does not watch children's programmes as she did before and refuses to go to her room on her own. She was adopted from abroad at the age of 9 months and there has been no concern about her. She can be very hyperactive and can take a long time to go to sleep. Cataract affects both of her eyes and is worse on the right. There are no other dysmorphic features. She can speak her natural parents' language, but is still immature and only can say a few single words. She walks with her head tilted to the left and looks down most of the time. The results from the CNS and another systemic examination are unremarkable. She was seen by an ophthalmologist, who confirmed a diagnosis of cataract. The ophthalmologist noted that she has keratoconus.

Chromosomes	Normal karyotyping
Urine AAs and organic acids	Normal
Plasma AAs	Normal
Lactate	1.7 mmol/l
Ammonia	25 mmol/l
GAG	Normal
Cranial MRI	Normal
KUB US	Normal
MSU	
Protein	++
RBC	++
WCC	Negative
Organism	Negative
Nitrite	Negative
pH	6.0

1. What one other clinical test should be carried out?
   - a Visual field
   - b BP
   - c Hearing test
   - d Examine fundi
   - e Wood light test
   - f Colour vision test
2. What is the diagnosis?
   - a Congenital cataract
   - b Congenital infection
   - c Retinoblastoma
   - d Down syndrome
   - e Goldenhar syndrome
   - f Stickler–Marshall syndrome

g   Lowe syndrome
h   Alport syndrome

Case 72

An ambulance crew brought a 14-year-old girl to A&E accompanied by her grandmother. The girl had a history of severe headache, slurred speech, and said she couldn't see. She said that the light was hurting her eyes and she was finding it very difficult to speak. The headache started first and then she could not move her left arm and leg. There is no family history of any illnesses and she is a fit and healthy girl. She is staying with her grandmother over the half-term holiday for a few days. She was visiting a friend the night before. She does not smoke or drink alcohol. Her older brother joined the Army. Her two younger siblings are healthy. She is irritable and opens her eyes on command. There is evidence of right facial nerve palsy. She is not able to move her left arm and leg. The results of other examinations are normal. The fundi are very clear and there is no evidence of papilloedema. She said her headache is very bad on the right-hand side. Her grandmother phoned the girl's mother and asked her whether her daughter was taking any medication. She has been taking medicine for headaches for the last 2 months. A cranial CT scan shows no abnormalities, even with contrast. Her U&Es, LFT, FBC, gases, and clotting are normal. An LP was carried out and shows no evidence of meningitis, cells or blood. Blood was sent for HSV PCR. She was treated with antibiotics and aciclovir, which was stopped after 5 days, after all results were back to normal. A cranial MRI scan and EEG were both reported as normal. Her grandmother also mentioned that her other daughter suffers from similar episodes. She was diagnosed as having transient hemiplegia and was not given any medication. This girl recovered very quickly and was discharged home after 10 days.

1. What are four differential diagnoses?
    a   Subarachnoid haemorrhage
    b   Meningoencephalitis
    c   Encephalitis
    d   Meningitis
    e   Substance abuse
    f   Migraine attack
    g   Cerebral infarct
2. What are the diagnoses?
    a   Alternating hemiplegia syndrome
    b   Familial hemiplegic migraine
    c   Classical migraine
    d   Paroxysmal vertigo
    e   Cerebral infarct

Case 73

A 2-year-old boy presented with a history of FTT and weight below the 3rd centile. He was born at term with no neonatal problems apart from jaundice, which required phototherapy. He was breast-fed for 6 months then changed to formula and then to high-energy formula, which did not help. At the time of presentation he is having solids plus two bottles (8 oz) of milk every day. His mother is concerned about the number of nappies she uses per day (4–6 nappies/day). Otherwise he is happy in himself. He is very easily bruised and in the last 6 months it has taken him a long time to stop bleeding if started. He also has a lot of falls, is not able to run and is described by his mother as a 'wobbly child and clumsy'. He has a brother, aged 5, who is healthy, as are both parents. He looks very thin, walks with a wide base gait and falls every fifth step. There is reduced tone in his limbs and the reflexes in his lower limbs are difficult to elicit. His response to pain in his lower limbs is not as good as for the rest of his body. He has difficulty in recognising pictures and colours.

There is no hepatosplenomegaly, or skin rashes. The fundi are normal and he is still in nappies. The test results are:

Hb	7.9 g/dl
WCC	11.6×10^9/l
PLT	350×10^9/l
INR	1.7
PTT	55 s
PT	90 s
TT	60 s
ESR	< 2 mm/hour
Ferritin	6
Blood film	Shows abnormal red blood cells which are not blast cells

1. What is the most likely diagnosis?
   a   Wilson disease
   b   Cystic fibrosis
   c   Schwachman syndrome
   d   Abetalipoproteinaemia
   e   Coeliac disease
   f   Inflammatory bowel disease
   g   Cows' milk protein intolerance

2. Which two other investigations are needed to establish the diagnosis?
   a   Sweat test
   b   Stool elastasis
   c   Stool fat
   d   Serum cholesterol level
   e   Serum triglyceride level
   f   Endomyseal antibodies
   g   Stool for reducing substances
   h   Upper and lower GIT endoscopy with biopsy
   i   Chest X-ray
   j   Caeruloplasmin level
   k   Urine for reducing substances
   l   Serum alpha-fetoprotein

3. Which two complications are associated with this condition?
   a Meconium ileus equivalent
   b Rickets
   c Retinitis pigmentosa
   d Short stature
   e Diabetes mellitus
   f Spastic quadriplegia
   g GIT lymphoma
   h Immune deficiency
   i Chronic lung disease

Case 74

A 3-week-old baby presented with a history of vomiting, diarrhoea, failure to regain birthweight, and persistent jaundice. He was born at term during a normal pregnancy and the scan at 34 weeks of gestation was normal. Early during the booking scan, there was a suggestion of pelvic renal dilatations (PRD) of 9 mm on the right. He has been breast-fed since birth; there is always plenty of milk and he is always hungry. Trial of top-up has failed, as he vomited more frequently. There is no family history of any illnesses and both parents are healthy. His liver is 3 cm below the costal margin and he looks jaundiced and lethargic. His stool colour is yellow and his urine is clear. His capillary refill time is 4 s, BP 40/50 mmHg and HR 130 b.p.m., with an RR of 35/min. His blood glucose level is 2.2 mmol/l and the Sat in air level is 90%. He is not crying. He was assessed and given 20 ml/kg of 0.9% NaCl over 30 min and i.v. ceftriaxone was given. O$_2$ was given at 3 L/m via a facemask with a reservoir, and his Sat is 97%, his CRT is now 3 s, BP 60/40 mmHg and HR 130 b.p.m. His blood culture detected *Escherichia coli*, which was treated successfully, but he returned 2 weeks later with jaundice, lethargy vomiting and was not feeding. An examination at the time showed a large liver measuring 4 cm below the right costal margin. The baby looks pale with corneal haziness and an absent red reflex. He was admitted for investigation, which shows that he is anaemic, and his urine is positive for sugar as well as protein. Blood and urine cultures were negative. His weight is on the 3rd centile and his height is on the 25th centile. He was treated i.v. fluids and his feeding was stopped but he continues to vomit. A TORCH screen test was negative, as was hepatitis serology. I.v. fluid was stopped and he was sent home after 48 hours. After 2 days, he was admitted with severe dehydration as he had not stopped vomiting since he was discharged 2 days before. Other test results are:

Na	135 mmol/l
K	3.6 mmol/l
U	7 mmol/l
Cr	70 mmol/l
PTT	130 s
PT	60 s

INR	1.9
Alb	22 g/l
Conjugated bilirubin	220 µmol/l

Urine

γGT	460 IU/l
ALT	50 IU/l
Alk. Ph	350 IU/l
Bill	250 µmol/l
Blood glucose	2.3 mmol/l
Protein	Positive
AAs	Positive
Blood	Negative
pH	6.1
MSU	Glucose positive

1. What other three tests are required to confirm the diagnosis?
   - a   LP
   - b   Abdominal US
   - c   Urine for reducing substances
   - d   Galactose-1-phosphate test (gal-1-p)
   - e   IgM for rubella
   - f   Viral serology
   - g   Plasma AAs
   - h   Urine organic acids
   - i   ABG
   - j   Lactate level
   - k   RBC enzyme assay for gal-1-p uridyltransferase (GUT)
2. What are the most likely diagnoses?
   - a   Septicaemia
   - b   Biliary atresia
   - c   Galactosaemia
   - d   Hypothyroidism
   - e   Congenital rubella infection
   - f   Viral hepatitis
   - g   Inborn error of metabolism
   - h   Lactose intolerance

Case 75

In the last 3 weeks, a 4-year-old boy has complained that he was not able to stand up from a sitting position. He has also put on a lot of weight and has a short temper. He was born at term to unrelated parents and had no neonatal problems. He was admitted at the age of 18 months with a history of possible seizures and his blood sugar at the time was 3 mmol/l. The fasting blood sugar for an overnight stay in hospital was 4.3 mmol/l. His height is on the 3rd centile and his weight on the > 97th centile. He feels he cannot go swimming as others have teased him for the skin striae on his flanks and legs. Sometimes he complains of headaches and cramps in his legs if he walk or plays for a considerable amount of time. He snores whilst sleeping and sometimes will make loud noises, as if he has something stuck in his throat. His blood pressure is 110/75 mmHg. Multiple striae are present with trunkal obesity. The results of a CNS examination are normal and there is no organomegaly. The CVS and genitalia are normal. A fundi examination was carried out by an ophthalmologist and reported as normal. He is not taking any medication. Other test results are:

Glu	4.2 mmol/l
ACTH	600 IU/l
Cortisol	200 mU/l (and midnight) 240 mU/l
FSH	3.5 mU/l
Urinary cortisol level	Normal
Short dexamethasone suppression test (overnight)	Equivocal

1. What is the possible cause?
   a   Pituitary ACTH hypersecretion (Cushing's disease)
   b   Malignant adrenal tumour
   c   Ectopic ACTH secretion
   d   Iatrogenic Cushing syndrome
2. Which single test would support the diagnosis?
   a   Short Synacthen test
   b   Glucagon test
   c   A 2-day low-dose dexamethasone-suppression test
   d   MRI of brain
   e   Abdominal CT
   f   Adrenal iodocholesterol scintigraphy

Case 76

A 3-year-old boy presented with a history of tiredness, vomiting and jaundice. He is known to have a blood disorder, which he receives treatment for with regular injections. He has also had six blood transfusions in the last 2 years. The last transfusion was given 3 weeks ago following an operation on his right knee to correct joint deformity. His sister, aged 9 years, is healthy, as is his younger brother. He was diagnosed with the blood disorder at the age of 3 months, when he presented with a large bruise on his leg. He looks ill with an HR of 110 b.p.m. and a BP of 90/65 mmHg. His sclerae are yellow and his liver measures 3 cm below the costal margin and has smooth edges. There is slight cervical lymphadenopathy on both sides of the neck and axilla. He has lost weight and has not been eating for the last 3 days, only taking water or juice. His joints are clear except the right knee, which is still sore, and he is not able to bend it. He can walk without difficulty but feels tired. He is fully immunised and there is no family history of illness. His mother is adopted and his father is healthy. His FBC and U&Es levels are normal. The abdominal US shows a large, smooth liver. His urine shows bilirubin but no red cells or leukocytes. The blood film shows spherocytes and target cells only. His liver function is abnormal, with conjugated and unconjugated hyperbilirubinaemia. Other test results are:

INR	1.7
PTT	120 s
VIIIc	> 30%
HIV antibody test	Negative

1. Which other three tests should be carried out?
   - a Liver biopsy
   - b Hepatitis C serology
   - c Hepatitis A serology
   - d Hepatitis B serology
   - e CMV serology
   - f AAs
   - g Caeruloplasmin level
   - h Upper GIT endoscopy
2. What are the three most likely diagnoses in order?
   - a Hepatitis C
   - b Hepatitis B
   - c Haemolytic anaemia
   - d Haemosiderosis
   - e Haemoglobinopathies
   - f Portal hypertension
   - g HIV infection
   - h Metabolic disease
   - i Liver cirrhosis

Case 77

A 3-year-old girl presented with limb pain and fever. She is pointing to her right thigh and finds it difficult to walk long distances. Recently she has started to cry whenever she is made to walk from home to nursery, which is about 1 mile from home. Her mother also commented that she has lost her colour and energy. She had a febrile illness 2 weeks ago, but no cause was found and her mother said she is still hot from time to time and becomes very irritable. She was admitted to hospital for further investigation. Her temperature rose to 37.5°C while she was asleep. By the morning, her left eye started to swell and she was treated for orbital cellulitis. There was no improvement with antibiotics and she was referred to an ophthalmologist, who diagnosed orbital cellulitis and advised that she be given a cranial CT scan. The scan showed soft-tissue swelling with erosion of sphenoidal bone around the left eye. An X-ray of the lower limbs shows no abnormality and a CXR was also normal. The blood culture came back as negative and 5 days of i.v. antibiotics were given without benefit. Her left eye is swollen and the ophthalmologist asked to see her again. Another cranial MRI scan was ordered, which was not very different from the previous CT scan carried out 3 days earlier. She cannot see with her left eye and analgesia controls the pain but she still has a temperature at night that reaches as high as 37.8°C. There is no organomegaly, joint swelling or painful joints. She is anaemic and her blood film was reported by a haematologist as hypochromic/normocytic with no blast cells. The results of a connective-tissue screen were negative and the ESR was only 10 mm/hour.

1. What one investigation is likely to be helpful?
   a   Bone marrow aspiration
   b   Bone scan
   c   White cell scan
   d   Abdominal MRI scan
   e   Barium swallow
   f   MRA and venogram
   g   Chest spiral CT

The test, which was carried out, reported abnormal cells but not lymphoblasts or myeloblast. Leukaemia was ruled out, as was Hodgkin's disease. Further tests were arranged at a regional centre.

2. Which other three tests are needed to confirm the diagnosis?
   a   Lesional biopsy
   b   Urinary VMA
   c   MIBG scan
   d   Abdominal US
   e   Karyotyping
   f   LP for TB screen
   g   VEP
   h   Mantoux test
3. What is the most likely diagnosis?

Case 78

A girl developed pubic hair and her breasts started to develop when she was only 6 years old. This started 2 months ago and her mother was assured that this may be due to the girl's being overweight, as she weighed 24 kg at that time. Her mother was very worried. The girl has not experienced any other symptoms. Her older sister started puberty at the age of 11 years and her mother at the age of 12. She is not taking medication and has no other problems. Her breasts and pubic hair are at Tanner stage 3. There are a few axillary hairs and no abdominal masses. Her FBC, U&Es, and LFT are all normal. The bone age is 9 years and a cranial MRI is normal. An abdominal US shows a multicystic ovarian appearance.

1. Which other investigations should be carried out?
   a   FSH level
   b   LH level

    c   Gonadotrophin profile overnight
    d   Testosterone level
    e   Oestradiol level
    f   Urine 17 hydroxyprogesterone level
    g   Chromosomes
    h   Bone X-ray
    i   Upper and lower GIT endoscopy
    j   Short Synacthen test
    k   Glucagon test
    l   Insulin-stimulation test
    m   Luteinising hormone-releasing hormone (LHRH) stimulation test
    n   Exercise test
2. What are the differential diagnoses?
    a   Central precocious puberty
    b   Gonadotrophin-independent precocious puberty
    c   Thyroid disease
    d   Congenital adrenal hyperplasia
    e   Intersex
    f   Premature thelarche
    g   Ovarian cyst
    h   Polycystic ovary syndrome

Case 79

A 13-year-old girl presented with a history of excess weight, intermittent headache and striae on the thighs. She also complained of tiredness and is not able to concentrate at school. She said she can not go out any more as children in the street call her names. Her puberty has not started yet and she is not worried about that, as there are two girls in her class who haven't started yet. She is not the shortest in her class. Her mother started her period at the age of 13. She finds it difficult to read because this sometimes causes her to have a headache. She sustained an injury to the left side of her head 2 days ago as she said she could not see the angle of a corner of the wall at school. Her optician gave her glasses for reading, which sometimes helps.

Her BP is 100/60 mmHg and HR 65 b.p.m. All cranial nerves are intact and fundi show a blurred right disc margin on the right side, which was confirmed by the ophthalmologist. There is a haematoma on the side of her head as a result of the injury 2 days ago. She can only read with reading glasses. Her headaches responded partially to paracetamol. She was admitted for overnight observation. The rest of the results from a CNS examination are unremarkable. Other test results are:

FBC, U&Es and LFT   Normal
MSU   No red or white cells

1. Which two abnormalities are visible on her SXR?

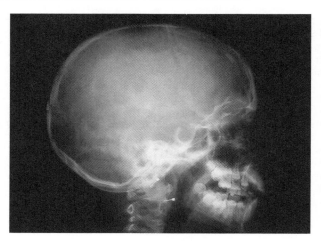

2. What one bedside test should be carried out?
3. Which four other tests are required to confirm the diagnosis?
4. What is the prognosis?

Case 80

A 3-month-old infant presented with a history of seizures in the early morning. His mother woke up after she heard banging noises in his cot. She found him with all of his limbs shaking. He stopped within 2 minutes and by the time the ambulance crew arrived he started moving his limbs and opened his eyes. A blood glucose test was carried out and showed that his glucose level was 1 mmol/l. He was given milk and taken to the hospital. On arrival he is still drowsy. His BM is 2.3 after 60 ml of milk. He was given another feed, which he did not take and went to sleep. Five minutes later he had apnoea, which required bagging and an anaesthetist was called for elective intubation. Blood was sent and 20 ml of 0.9% NaCl was given. He was seen in the Outpatient Department at 1 week of age with hypotonia, and a follow-up appointment was arranged with a neurologist. His tests for FBC, U&Es and TFT were all normal. A urine test did not show ketones, blood or protein. His parents lost a female child at the age of 2 months to sudden infant death syndrome (SIDS). The results of the blood, CSF lactate and glycine tests are normal. The NH_4 level was 150 mmol/l (40–70 mmol/l). The plasma AAs show a high level of glycine and methylmalonate.

ALT	280 IU/l
Alk. Ph	600 IU/l
γGT	130 IU/l
Alb	32 g/l

Total protein	70 g/l
Urine	
Ketones	Negative
WCC	< 10
Glu	Negative
Pro	Negative
Anion gap	> 20
Arterial gas	
Ph	7.23
PCO_2	3.4 kpa
PO_2	7.3 kpa
HCO_3	12
Be	−13
Blood culture	Negative
Serum urate	Normal
Transferrin level	Normal

1. List four other investigations that should be carried out on this patient?
   a   Mass spectroscopy for acetylglycine in urine and blood
   b   Liver biopsy
   c   WCC enzyme assay
   d   Cultured skin fibroblast
   e   Cranial MRI
   f   Echocardiography
   g   EMG
2. What are the two most likely diagnoses in order?
   a   Septicaemia
   b   Viral infection
   c   Medium-chain acetyl-CoA dehydrogenase deficiency (MCAD)
   d   Lactic acidosis
   e   Non-ketotic hyperglycinaemia
   f   Fatty acid oxidation defect
   g   Glycogen storage disease
   h   Mitochondrial disease

ANSWERS 71–80

Case 71

1. c   Hearing test
2. h   Alport syndrome

Hereditary nephritis (Alport syndrome)

The mode of inheritance varies among affected families and is more severe in males than females. The gene is located on the X chromosome. It is characterised by progressive nephritic haematuria, sensorineural deafness and ocular abnormalities in the form of cataract and anterior lenticonus. The pathology on renal biopsy will show focal mesangial hypercellularity with progressive glomerular sclerosis, tubular atrophy, and interstitial inflammation and foam cells. It is usually asymptomatic in childhood, but some members of an affected family may show progressive haematuria and proteinuria. In the second decade of life it will become worse, with worsened haematuria, proteinuria and renal failure. The deafness is initially high frequency and progressive, and later becomes profound. Diagnosis can be made on histological examination from renal biopsy. There is no treatment available other than dialysis and renal transplant if the patient progresses to chronic renal failure.

Case 72

1. d   Meningitis
   c   Encephalitis
   g   Cerebral infarct
   f   Migrainous attack
2. b   Familial hemiplegic migraine

Familial hemiplegic migraine

This is characterised by a sudden onset of headache with hemiplegia. It is usually accompanied by a neurological deficit during the attack or after such as in seventh nerve palsy. Patients may experience other symptoms such as nausea, vomiting, and weakness or lethargy. The attacks may last several hours to a few days, but are usually only a few hours' duration and the patient is usually then back to normal. Other members of the family are often affected and it may occur at any age. There are longer gaps between each attack and most patients grow out of it. If a family history is clear, no further investigation is needed, but if there is doubt then a full assessment of the risk of stroke in children is needed after discussion with a specialist in this field.

Case 73

1. d   Abetalipoproteinaemia
2. d   Serum cholesterol level
   e   Serum triglyceride level
3. c   Retinitis pigmentosa
   b   Rickets

Abetalipoproteinaemia

This is a disorder of lipid metabolism that is transmitted as an autosomal recessive trait with apolipoprotein B missing from the serum. Apolipoprotein B is essential for the synthesis of low-density and very-low-density lipoproteins. There will be malabsorption of fat as well as of vitamins A, E, and K. FTT is the commonest presentation in this group. Affected individuals pass a large volume of stool and show developmental delay. Ataxia develops in one-third of children in the first 10 years of life and in all by the second decade. There will be dysmetria, gait disturbances, and ataxia that progress until the third decade and then stop. The tendon reflexes will be lost by the age of 5 years and the proprioception sensation is lost in the hands and feet; this is as a result of demyelination of peripheral nerves and posterior columns. Retinitis pigmentosa is not a constant feature and can develop later in the first decade. Acanthocytes are the hallmark of abetalipoproteinaemia and other lipoprotein deficiencies. About 50–70% of erythrocytes will transform to acanthocytes. Anaemia in the form of microcytic/hypochromic anaemia due to malabsorption of iron is a common feature. The cholesterol and triclyceride levels are reduced. The absence of plasma apolipoprotein is diagnostic. A low-fat diet with vitamin supplements of A, E, and K should be given to prevent the neurological symptoms and reverse the neuropathy and myopathy.

Case 74

1. c   Urine for reducing substances
    d   Gal-1-p test
    k   RBC enzyme assay for gal-1-p uridyltransferase (GUT)
2. c   Galactosaemia

Galactosaemia

This is a metabolic disorder due to inborn errors of lactose metabolism. The commonest form, which may lead to mental retardation, is due to GUT deficiency. The newborn looks normal at birth but will soon develop hypoglycaemia after introduction of feed. Then the child fails to thrive and has vomiting, diarrhoea, and hepatomegaly. Cataracts may be present earlier, but not in all patients. Newborns with galactosaemia can become very sick and behave as if they have sepsis. No one knows why these babies develop *E. coli* sepsis; there seems to be an association between *E. coli* and galactosaemia. The presentation can be with prolonged jaundice and poor weight gain. Urine should be tested for reducing substances; Clinitest tablets will be positive for glucose but Clinistix will be negative. The gal-1-p test is markedly elevated, even in cord blood, and early detection can be made in high-risk groups in infants. Enzyme assay can be carried out for fibroblasts, chorionic villi and RBCs, but a galactose tolerance test should not be performed. Fatty infiltration and fibrosis occur in the liver; this can be seen on biopsy. In severe forms, the poor condition of the affected individual can be dramatic, with liver failure and a biochemical finding of Fanconi syndrome. If this condition is not treated, then FTT and sepsis with mental and behavioural problems will arise. Sometimes this condition can present simply as FTT and cataract, if the enzyme deficiency is minimal. A galactose-free diet for life is the treatment, but even so some children may develop complications. Dyspraxic speech is present in 50% of patients and hypogonadotrophic hypogonadism with ovarian failure and often sterility occurs in 80% of females.

Case 75

1.   a   Pituitary ACTH hypersecretion (Cushing's disease)
2.   c   2-day low-dose dexamethasone-suppression test

Cushing's disease

This disease is mainly caused by pituitary adenomas, which can be very small – 2–10 mm in size – and can be detected by contrast-enhanced pituitary MRI. The physical features do not differ from those of Cushing syndrome. These features are a result of advanced Cushing's disease. The signs – central obesity, moon facies, hirsutism, facial flushing, striae, muscular weakness (proximal), back pain, a buffalo hump and psychological disturbances – are all features of Cushing syndrome and advanced disease. Growth arrest is another feature and could be one of the earlier signs. Obesity in children with Cushing disease is different from obesity in children with Cushing syndrome. In Cushing disease it is generalised, with a buffalo hump having developed earlier, while in Cushing syndrome it will be central and the buffalo hump will develop later. Cushing's disease usually indicates a primary problem in the pituitary gland rather than something else. Surgical removal of pituitary microadenoma will result in a normal circadian rhythm, and ACTH and cortisol levels will return to normal. Cortisol will be easily suppressed by a low dose of dexamethasone. Cyproheptadine has no effect in paediatric patients, although good results have been obtained in adults with Cushing's disease when surgery is not the best option. Removal of the dermal glands will eliminate the physiological feedback inhibition mechanism of the pituitary. Low- and high-dose dexamethasone-suppression tests can be useful. This test can be done over 6 days, and collection of samples at different times will help to determine whether or not obesity is due to Cushing disease. Blood should be collected at 8.00 a.m. and 8.00 p.m. each day, as well as a 24-hour urine collection. In patients with exogenous obesity, or other non-Cushing disorders, cortisol, ACTH and urinary steroids will be suppressed by a low dose of dexamethasone. Patients with adrenal adenoma, adrenal carcinoma or ectopic ACTH secretion will have values relatively insensitive to both the low- and high-dose dexamethasone-suppression tests. Patients with Cushing's disease classically respond to a high but not low dose of dexamethasone by suppression of ACTH, cortisol and urinary steroids.

Case 76

1.   b, d Hepatitis serology for B and C
      a   Liver biopsy
2.   a, b Viral hepatitis B or C

g   HIV
d   Haemosiderosis

Viral hepatitis in children

This is characterised by hepatic inflammation and dysfunction, which includes hyperbilirubinaemia, an abnormal liver function test and dark yellow urine. There are elevations in serum aspartate aminotransferase, alkaline phosphatase, and gamma-glutamyltransferase. Other LFT functions are within normal values unless hepatitis becomes chronic. Very rarely, infants may have bleeding problems and the INR will be high; in this instance, vitamin K should be given. There are many causes of extra- and intrahepatic disorders causing hepatitis. Congenital infections, metabolic disorders, and biliary atresia may be the most frequent causes of hepatitis in infancy. Viral hepatitis in infancy may be due to CMV, EBV, rubella, varicella zoster, hepatitis A,B, non-A and non-B, coxsackie virus, HSV, ECHO virus, and adenovirus. Prolonged jaundice or abnormal liver function in infants will prompt investigators to find the cause. A stool sample should be sent for pigment testing. A clotted sample should be sent for virology testing (specific IgM). Abdominal US will help to rule out biliary tract abnormalities. Urine should be tested for reducing substances and a thyroid function test should be performed without delay. A liver biopsy is not indicated in viral hepatitis, but may be for other hepatitis. Hepatomegaly, which can be tender, smooth and firm, can be associated with viral hepatitis. The congenital or acquired viral infection will have a different prognosis, and advice from a hepatologist should be obtained.

Case 77

1.   a, Bone marrow aspiration
2.   a, Lesional biopsy
     b, Urinary VMA
     c, MIBG scan
3.   Neuroblastoma

Neuroblastoma

This arises from primordial neural crest cells of the sympathetic and occasionally parasympathetic nervous system. It is usually presented as an abdominal mass with other metastasis. The abdominal mass often crosses the midline, and features of bone marrow infiltration such as anaemia, thrombocytopenia, bruising, fever, lethargy and irritability are present. Adrenal glands are the commonest site of origin. Localised disease is most likely to occur in the neck or less commonly in pelvis or bone. Bone disease will cause very deep, uncomfortable pain. Most abdominal tumours will be metastasised at the time of diagnosis to bone, skin, liver and the CNS. Proptosis or periorbital swellings or bruising are characteristic features of a tumour within the orbit or sphenoidal bone. Spinal tumours may cause cord compression at any level of the spinal cord. The presence of high levels of catecholamines in the body will not cause high blood pressure. It may also present as acute cerebellar ataxia with rapid eye movement. Unilateral Horner syndrome may be due to cervical chain disease. Diagnosis can be confirmed by biopsy from the mass or bony lesions. Bone marrow aspiration is important to exclude metastasis and diagnosis. Imaging is important to find out more about the nature of the disease and help in staging. MRI, CT and CXR are all helpful. MIBG scans will help to localise bone involvement, this is a good marker. The measurement of urinary VMA, and HVA is vital in diagnosis as well as in evaluating response to treatment, and should be done by a 24-hour urinary collection test. The prognosis is very good for the localised disease but not for the advanced form. Good prognostic features include age < 1 year stage 1,2 and 4S disease, primary neck and thorax mass, and low serum ferritin level. Poor prognostic features include age > 1 year, abdominal mass, high ferritin level, and stages 3 and 4 disease.

Case 78

1. a,b FSH and LH levels
   e   Oestradiol level
   f   Urine 17- hydroxyprogesterone level
   d   Testosterone level
   k   Glucagon test
   m   LHRH stimulation test
   g   Chromosomes study
2. d   Congenital adrenal hyperplasia
   a   Central precocious puberty

Precocious puberty

Precocious puberty is a recognised complication of congenital adrenal hyperplasia in boys with 21-hydroxylase or 11-beta-hydroxylase deficiency. Boys who did not develop a salt-losing crisis during the neonatal or infantile period may present with precocious puberty (genital and pubic hair growth with normal testicular size). The height velocity and muscle bulk are increased with bone age, and may be advanced without achieving the optimum adult height.

Central precocious puberty in a small proportion of girls may be due to CNS tumours (chiasmatic/hypothalamic gliomas, astrocytoma, pineal tumours and cysts, astrocytoma, ependymoma, and pituitary adenoma), hydrocephalus, NFI, post-trauma head injuries, septo-optic dysplasia, hypothalamic hamartoma, and post-encephalitis or meningitis. The endocrine and physical events happen in the same way as for normal puberty. McCune–Albright syndrome, untreated hypothyroidism, and adrenal tumours will lead to precocious puberty. GnRh analogues are the first choice of treatment in central precocious puberty. For most individuals, the problem is self-limiting, with normal reproductive function.

Case 79

1. Large pituitary fossa
   Calcification of pituitary gland
2. Visual fields
3. Cranial MRI
   Random hormonal assay (GH, cortisol, TFT, FSH, LH)
   Serum and urine osmolality
   U&Es
4. Poor

Clinical presentation of intracranial lesions

There are many lesions arising from the hypothalamus, pituitary stalk, anterior pituitary, posterior pituitary, and pineal, which may affect growth. A GH-secreting tumour will cause acromegaly, which leads to gigantism, characterised by constantly raised GH, raised insulin-like growth factor I (IGF-I), and paradoxical response to glucagon-loading dose and thyrotrophin-releasing hormone (TRH). The persistent elevation of GH on 24-hour serum collection is a diagnostic test for gigantism. A pineal tumour and hypothalamic hamartomas will cause precocious puberty. Retention of growth due to prolactin-secreting tumours can be associated with craniopharyngiomas and other tumours. Cushing's disease, secondary to hypersecreting pituitary adenoma, is also associated with short stature. Any pituitary tumour may cause delay in sexual maturation. Craniopharyngiomas typically produce sexual infantilism and dystrophic adiposity. Tumours in the region of the sella turcica and suprasellar region can produce problems with vision. Bitemporal hemianopia is caused by suprasellar lesions, and loss of vision can occur if it affects the optic tract or nerve. A pineal tumour will cause problems with accommodation, difficulty with upward gaze, poor convergence and nystagmus. Blocking one or both foramina of Monro can lead to obstructive hydrocephalus, which may be caused by any lesion in the pituitary fossa, extending to the third ventricle. Increased intracranial pressure can be caused by any tumour growing from the pituitary fossa.

Case 80

1. a   Mass spectroscopy for acetyl-glycine in urine and blood
   b   Liver biopsy
   c   WCC enzyme assay
   d   Cultured skin fibroblast
2. c   MCAD
   f   Fatty acid oxidation defect

Methylmalonic acidaemia (MCAD)

The commonest enzyme deficiency in this group is mutase, which will lead to accumulation of propionyl CoA, propionic acid and methylmalonic acid and cause hyperglycinaemia and hyperammonaemia. It is transmitted as an autosomal recessive disorder in all groups causing MCAD. The child appears to be normal at birth, but symptoms start to appear in the first week in almost all babies with mutase deficiency. The baby will be lethargic, fail to gain weight, vomit, be dehydrated, and have hypotonia and respiratory distress after initiation of a protein feed. There will leukopenia, thrombocytopenia, and anaemia in the majority of cases, and it will mimic sepsis. CNS bleeding may occur as a result of the illness. The child will be acidotic and mainly metabolic with ketoses, hyperglycinaemia, and hyperammonaemia. Tests on plasma and urine AAs will show a high level of methylmalonate. A tissue fibroblast culture will detect specific enzyme deficiency. Supportive treatment and vitamin B_{12}, correcting acidosis with protein restriction to 1–1.5 g/kg/d, will help in many cases. L-Carnitine will reduce the ketogenesis in response to fasting. The prognosis is poor in mutase deficiency, and affected babies die within the first 2 months of life.

Case 81

An 11-year-old boy presented with a petechial rash and one bruise on his left arm. The rashes started 2 days ago but he remained afebrile and asymptomatic. He was fighting with his brother when he got the bruise. He was expelled from school because of his aggressive behaviour. His mother said his lip colour has looked different in the last 2 weeks: paler. He has had no previous admissions to hospital and he is a healthy young boy. He lives with his mother and stepfather, two sisters aged 16 and 17 years and a brother aged 12, who has epilepsy and a learning difficulty. He likes contact sports and fishing. He looks pale and has no jaundice. No lymphadenopathy is present but there is a petechial rash everywhere, especially on his arms. There is one large bruise on his left upper arm and a few small ones on his legs. There is no organomegaly and his blood pressure is 100/60 mmHg. His mother is worried about meningitis and he has been rushed to the hospital after he refused to have i.m. antibiotics at the GP's surgery. The test results for LFT, U&Es, CRP and ESR are normal. The FBC is only able to do WCCs, which are 53,000 and the clotting profile was normal. The blood film was reported as abnormal with cells looking like blast cells.

1. Which other tests can be helpful in managing this child?
   a FBC
   b CXR
   c Blood film was reported as abnormal
   d Viral serology
   e ANA
   f Abdominal US
   g Urine for VMA
   h Blood culture
   i MSU
   j Lumbar puncture
   k Throat swab
   l Stool culture
   FBC shows WCC of 53 000, platelets 50, and Hb of 9.9 g/dl
2. What is the most likely diagnosis?
   a Septicaemia
   b Trauma
   c Haemophilia
   d Viral infection
   e Hodgkin's lymphoma
   f Neuroblastoma
   g ALL
   h Non-Hodgkin's lymphoma
   i Vitamin K deficiency
   j ITP
   k Henoch–Schönlein purpura
   l Aplastic anaemia

3. What should be the five steps of the initial management?
   a   i.v. antibiotics if febrile
   b   Platelet transfusion
   c   Packed red cell transfusion with negative CMV
   d   Hyperhydration
   e   Oral allopurinol
   f   Arrange for bone marrow aspirate
   g   Avoid transfusion if there is no mucous membrane bleeding
   h   Arrange for LP
   i   Oral steroids
   j   I.v. immunoglobulin
   k   Observe and give no treatment
   l   Arrange transfer to specialist unit

Case 82

At the age of 14 days, a baby boy started to have generalised seizures without any obvious reason. He had been fed and his mother went back to check on him and found his body shaking all over. His eyes were open and rolled backward and his face was also twitching, mainly around his mouth. This stopped within 3 min and when the paramedics arrived he started to fit again but this time it lasted more than 5 min and rectal diazepam was given (2.5 mg). He stopped but needed O_2, as his saturation level was not good. He was transferred to hospital and required another dose of rectal diazepam to stop his seizures, which had started again. He continued to have apnoea, which was then reversed after he was intubated and ventilated and given flumazenil. He was extubated as soon as he arrived at the PICU. He had two further episodes of apnoea 2 days later, which required bagging with intermittent positive-pressure ventilation (IPPV), and he recovered quickly. His tone became more spastic and he started arching his back. This all resolved apart from the spacticity in his limbs. He went home on nasogastric feeding and various tests were organised, including an MRI scan. He was reviewed 2 months later and was found to have a small head (< 3rd centile) and his weight was < 10th centile. He was still on anti-epileptic drugs (AED), which did not control his seizures, and is now on two drugs (sodium valproate and lamotrigine). He has increased tone in his lower limbs, very poor head control, and continues to be fed nasogastrically. His urine shows elevated levels of glycine/valine. He is neutropenic with normal LFT and U&Es levels. The EEG demonstrates burst suppression patterns, with some element of hypsarrhythmia. The cranial MRI scan shows brain atrophy and demyelination. Other test results include:

NH_4	60 mmol/l
CSF	
Protein	0.37 g/l
Glu	2.1 mmol/l (serum 4.3 mmol/l)
WCC	< 10
Lactate	1.7 mmol/l (serum 2.1 mmol/l)

Glycine   40
Glycine/pyruvate ratio   < 20

1. Which other tests may provide useful information?
   a   Sleep EEG
   b   Cranial MRI
   c   Urinary ketones
   d   White cell enzyme
   e   Transferrin level
   f   Fibroblast cell culture
   g   Very-long-chain fatty acids (VLCF) level
   h   Serum AAs
2. What is the most likely diagnosis?
   a   Urea cycle defect
   b   Organic acidaemia
   c   Glycogen storage disease
   d   Fatty acid oxidation defect
   e   Carbohydrate-deficient glycoprotein syndrome
   f   Non-ketotic hyperglycinaemia
   g   Neonatal encephalopathy
   h   Congenital infection

Case 83

A 2-week-old baby boy was admitted with a history of abnormal colour and drowsiness after abnormal movements in his arms and legs for 3 min. He is a poor feeder and has not yet regained his birth weight. He is the third child born to a family of Bangladeshi origin. Both of his siblings are healthy (and as babies were healthy) apart from having eczema. The family has lived in the UK for the last 5 years and they visit grandparents in Bangladesh once every year, but not this year. He was born during a normal vaginal delivery at hospital, with no early neonatal events. He was discharged home after 24 hours and his weight and height at birth were on the 50th centile. During this admission, the baby was jittery, sleepy and not interested in feeding. He was afebrile, with a HR of 130 b.p.m., a RR of 20/min, and an O_2 Sat level of 96% in air. He is totally breast-fed and his mother is keen for this to continue. He has no birthmarks and other systemic and general examinations show no abnormalities. His head US was reported as normal, and nasogastric tube (NGT) feeding was started. Other test results are:

Na	136 mmol/l
K	4.2 mmol/l
Urea	5.2mmol/l
Cr	55 mmol/l
Ca	1.60 mmol/l
Alb	33 g/l
Mg	0.63 mmol/l
pH	7.36
PCO_2	4.2 kPa

PO_2	9.5 kPa
Urine	Negative for blood, glucose and ketones
CRP	< 5
Blood culture	Negative

1. What is the single most important investigation?
    a   Lumbar puncture
    b   Full blood count
    c   Liver function test
    d   Coagulation screen
    e   CXR
    f   AXR
    g   Blood glucose
    h   Mother's serum calcium level

His plasma glucose level was 4.6 mmol/l even before the resuscitation fluid was given, and reached 5 mmol/l after.

2. What is the diagnosis?
    a   Seizures secondary to hypoglycaemia
    b   Seizures secondary to hypocalcaemia
    c   Seizures secondary to hypomagnesaemia
    d   Seizures secondary to sepsis
    e   Seizures secondary to inborn error of metabolism
3. What other investigations should be carried out on this child?
    a   Parathyroid hormone level
    b   Renal US
    c   Mother's parathyroid hormone level
    d   Mother's serum calcium level
    e   Cranial MRI scan
    f   Chromosomal study
    g   Serum ammonia
    h   Serum lactate
    i   Baby's alkaline phosphatase level
    j   Baby's vitamin D level

Case 84

A 2-year-old boy presented with right knee pain and was not able to walk. He is febrile and irritable, and not able to bear weight on his feet. He just sits on his mother's lap and does not smile or interact with other people. He has had more than five ear infections and one bout of gastroenteritis that required admission to hospital for 1 week. His sister is 4 years old and is healthy. There is no family history of any illness apart from his cousin, who is the same age and was admitted to hospital with a bad case of meningitis 2 months ago. The boy is thriving and has had all of his vaccinations. He had a chest infection 3 months ago that required i.v. antibiotics. A sweat test was carried out at the time and reported as normal. He failed to attend an outpatient appointment for further assessment and investigation. His right knee is swollen, red and hot. He is in pain and is not allowing anyone to touch his knee. His temperature is 38.5°C, his HR is 120 b.p.m. and his RR 18/min. His blood pressure was not tested and the CRT is < 2 s. There is a discharge from his right ear and he is on an antibiotic for this, which his mother does not know the name of. The chest and abdominal examination is unremarkable. Analgesia was given, his knee was examined by the orthopaedic team and a diagnosis of septic arthritis was made. Arrangements were made for a US to be carried out and it was noted that the knee may need to be drained later. Treatment with broad-spectrum antibiotics was commenced, with regular analgesia. A right-knee US shows only soft-tissue swelling with a high ESR and CRP. He was discharged home to complete a course of 10 days of i.v. antibiotics.

1. Which four other tests should be organised?
    a Bone scan
    b MRI scan of right knee
    c Ig level
    d Antibody for pertussis and Hib vaccine
    e CD19/20 markers
    f Bone marrow biopsy
    g Viral serology
    h Blood film
    i Urinary VMA
    j Lymphocyte subset
    k HIV test
    l White cell scan
2. What are the most likely diagnoses?
    a X-linked agammaglobulinaemia
    b Severe combined immune deficiency (SCID)
    c ALL
    d Neuroblastoma
    e Schwachman syndrome
    f SLE
    g Adenosine deaminase deficiency
    h AIDS

Case 85

A 7-year-old girl was admitted to a paediatric ward with a history of high temperature, back pain, and headache for the last 25 days. Her GP treated her for a UTI, even though the culture was negative. The back pain occurs mainly on L4 and L5. NSAIDs are helping to relieve her pain but it comes back as these wear off. Her father is originally from Malta and every summer the family spends 6 weeks in her grandparents' home there. Her grandfather lives on a farm with different animals, but mainly cattle. She is lethargic, feels weak and has muscle pain and headaches. She had fever for 3 days, 3 weeks ago and antibiotics were given for a sore throat. She has lost 4 kg in weight in the last 2 months. Her brother and parents are healthy. There is slight cervical lymphadenopathy on both sides, but no abnormality was found on general and systemic examination. She was admitted and overnight her temperature reached 39°C. She had profuse sweating and rigors. Her back pain is much improved with analgesia. She was started on broad-spectrum i.v. antibiotics, as her CRP was 230. A lumbar spine X-ray reported no abnormality. Mantoux tests of 1:10 000 and 1:1000 are negative. The sickle-cell screen and CXR were reported as normal but her abdominal US reported a spleen size of about 2 cm below the left costal margin. Other test results are:

Blood film	Lymphocytosis with normochromic, normocytic picture. No parasites seen
Haemoglobin electrophoresis	No evidence of thalassaemia or other haemoglobinopathies.
ECHO	No abnormalities
Leptospirosis/Lyme disease screen	Negative
Bone scan	Normal
ANA, rheumatoid factors, and DNA double strand (carried out by her GP)	Normal

1. What are the most likely diagnoses?
   a   Osteomyelitis
   b   Juvenile chronic arthritis (JCA)
   c   Ankylosing spondylitis
   d   Brucellosis
   e   Bone malignancy
   f   Tuberculosis
   g   Myositis
   h   Chronic viral infection
   i   Viral hepatitis
   j   Malaria
2. Which other one single test should you carry out?
   a   Hot spot biopsy
   b   Bone marrow biopsy
   c   White cell scan
   d   Lymph node biopsy
   e   *Brucella*-specific IgM titres
   f   Repeat blood film for malaria
   g   Gastric aspirate for mycobacteria
   h   Spinal MRI
   i   Thick blood film
   j   Hepatitis A,B, and C serology
   k   *Mycoplasma* titres
3. What is the treatment?

Case 86

A 14-year-old known asthmatic with a history of increasing wheezy episodes was seen in A&E. He was travelling by air and before landing he started having difficulty in breathing. He was given O_2 and 10 puffs of his inhaler. He improved a little and was then taken to a clinic in the airport, where he was treated twice with a nebuliser, which helped a lot. When he was seen in hospital, his RR was 25/min, Sat level 96% in air and HR 110 b.p.m., with a wheeze heard on auscultation. He was diagnosed as having asthma 2 years ago by his previous GP and he takes a regular inhaler, which he said most of the time he does not need. He is also under investigation for goitre. The thyroid gland is palpable, measures about 3 × 4 cm, and is soft and not nodular. There is no bruising or lymphadenopathy. He has expiratory wheezes and inspiratory stridor, which is worse when lying down. He required O_2 overnight for desaturation while he was sleeping. His thyroid function, FBC, ESR and blood film are reported as normal. Other test results are:

PEFR   300 l/min
Height   25th centile

1. What two abnormalities appear on the lung function test?

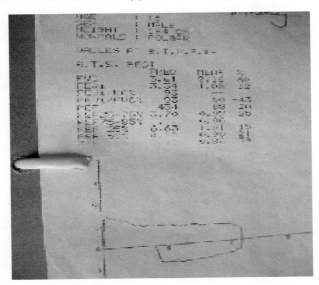

2. What two abnormalities appear on the CXR shown on the next page?
3. What are the two most immediately useful tests?
    a   Bone marrow aspirate
    b   Lateral CXR
    c   Spiral chest and abdominal CT
    d   Chest MRI
    e   Radioisotope scan
    f   Chest US

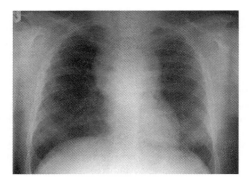

4. What are the three most likely diagnoses?
   a   T-cell lymphoma
   b   Thymoma
   c   Teratoma
   d   Thyroid gland enlargement
   e   Malignant thyroid gland carcinoma
   f   Bronchogenic cyst
   g   Lymphoma
   h   Neuroblastoma
5. What should the management plan be before he travels to his home?
   a   Blood transfusion
   b   Hyperhydration
   c   i.v. antibiotics
   d   Thyroxine replacement
   e   Allopurinol
   f   Oral hydrocortisone
   g   Intubation and ventilation
   h   Radiotherapy
   i   Start chemotherapy
   j   Blood karotyping and immunological and chemical studies
   k   Transfer to specialist unit
   l   Tissue biopsy from mediastinal mass
   m   Bone marrow biopsy
   n   Start dexamethasone after all investigations are carried out
   o   Save serum
   p   Repeat lung function test before travel

Case 87

A 10-year-old Afro-Caribbean girl presented with a history of inability to walk without muscle pain. Her problem started 3 months ago, when her eyes got swollen and she was treated as having periorbital cellulitis, which improved over 1 week but left erythema on her face.

She says she is tired most of the time and finds it very difficult to walk up stairs; she sometimes asks her 13-year-old brother to help her to go upstairs. She noticed that her knuckles become swollen from time to time and her skin pigmentation appears to be different in various places. She was diagnosed as having eczema and applies creams to her skin, which help, but it returns 2 weeks later. There are two lumps on her left elbow and she said these have been there for the last 3 months, following her fall on that elbow at school. She looks tired and has skin discoloration around her eyes. There is proximal muscle weakness in her limbs. All reflexes and cranial nerves are intact. Joint movement in her hands is not painful. There is no other abnormality. An X-ray of her ankle joints was reported as normal, as well as an eye examination. Blood tests on her renal and liver function are normal. The erythrocyte sedimentation rate (ESR) is 200 mm/hour. She says she cannot go to school as she finds it difficult to cope with the daily activity there. There is no extraocular muscle involvement and no evidence of petechial rash or joint thickening.

1. What is the most likely diagnosis?
    a   JCA
    b   SLE
    c   Dermatomyositis
    d   Polymyositis
    e   Myasthenia gravis
    f   Scleroderma
    g   Viral infection
2. Which five tests are the most useful?
    a   Thigh muscle MRI
    b   Muscle biopsy
    c   EMG
    d   CK
    e   LDH
    f   NCS
    g   Cranial MRI
    h   Slit lamp eye examination
    i   Viral serology
    j   DNA double strand
    k   ANA
    l   X-ray of right elbow
3. What should the management plan be?
    a   Oral steroids for 6 months
    b   i.v. steroids
    c   IVIG
    d   Azathioprine
    e   Methotrexate
    f   Physiotherapy
    g   Plasmapheresis
    h   Physiotherapy
    i   Occupational therapy

Case 88

A girl aged 3 years presents with diarrhoea, which has lasted for the past 2 months. She opens her bowel four times per day and sometimes more often. The stool is firmer in the morning and looser in the evening, which is consistent on a daily basis. There is no blood or mucus in her stool. She had gastroenteritis prior to this, which she recovered from, but then 2 weeks later this problem started. Her weight remains above the 25th centile and there has been no loss of weight over the last 3 months. Her mother said she complains every day of abdominal pain around lunchtime, which may last 30–60 min and has no relation to her food. When she is eating an apple or has cereal in the morning, her stool frequency is worse and she experiences more abdominal pain. Her stool often contains undigested food. Her parents travel twice each year to South America for a holiday and to see family. She has no other problems and both her brothers and parents are healthy. There is no organomegaly or skin problem. The results of a systemic examination were normal and her weight and height are on the 25th centile. A stool culture was taken for bacteria, cysts, and virology, and there is no parasite or bacteria growth. She is not anaemic and an abdominal US was reported as normal. Her urine is clear and there was no bacterial growth after 48 hours.

A test on a stool sample for reducing substances was negative. FBC, LFT, amylase, TFT, Ig, and culture from three fresh stools were reported as normal. Endomyseal antibodies are negative and antiglidan IgA antibodies are weakly positive.

1. What is the diagnosis?
    a   Coeliac disease
    b   Infective diarrhoea
    c   Crohn's disease
    d   Ulcerative colitis
    e   Eosinophilic colitis
    f   Cows' milk (CMPI) protein intolerance
    g   Lactose intolerance
    h   Toddler's diarrhoea
    i   Cystic fibrosis
2. Which other tests may help the diagnosis?
    a   Barium swallow and follow-through
    b   Abdominal US
    c   Upper GIT endoscopy
    d   Lower GIT endoscopy
    e   Nothing
    f   Repeat stool for reducing substances
    g   Sweat test
    h   Stool for fat

Case 89

A 6-month-old boy was born by ELSCS for fetal distress. There was thick meconium, which required suction and IPPV, and admission to the neonatal unit for 3 days. His O_2 requirement in the first 24 hours was 30% via a head box, then it improved. His CXR shows evidence of small granulation and a fluffy shadow in the lung fields. He was discharged home after 7 days, and on follow-up at the age of 3 months he was thriving well. His OFC at birth was 38 cm, and he had syndactyly, a flat nasal bridge and a birth mark on his right shoulder. His OFC was 42 cm at 3 months and 50 cm at 6 months. The father's OFC is 57 and his mother's is 52 cm. His fontanelle is widely open with hypertelorism, and skull sutures are mildly open. He can sit with support and is making a lot of noises. He can roll from back to front and front to back. He changes objects from one hand to the other and has started to point. He smiled at the age of 8 weeks and had good head control at the age of 3 months. His grandmother had syndactyly and there are no other illnesses in the family. He is the only child in the family and both parents are healthy.

1.   What abnormality is visible on the cranial CT?

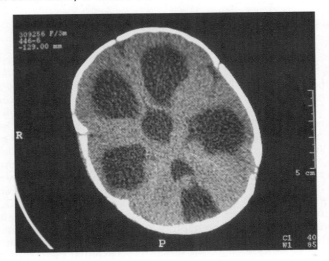

a   Dilated lateral ventricles
b   Dilated third ventricles
c   Dilated fourth ventricle
d   External hydrocephalus
e   Subdural haemorrhage

    f   Cranial synostosis
    g   Bulky choroid plexus
    h   Grey matter calcified lesions

2. What is the most likely diagnosis?
    a   Non-communicating hydrocephalus
    b   Hydrocephalus secondary to plexiform papilloma
    c   Hydrocephalus secondary to congenital infection
    d   Communicating hydrocephalus
    e   Choroid plexus papilloma
    f   Interventricular tumour
    g   Hydrocephalus secondary to IVH
    h   Hydrocephalus secondary to HIE

3. How should this child be managed?
    a   Eye examination
    b   TORCH screen
    c   Chromosomal analysis
    d   Refer to neurosurgeon
    e   Refer to paediatric neurologist
    f   Cranial CT on father
    g   Urinary organic acids

Case 90

A 13-year-old boy presented with a history of collapse after a game of football with his friends. During the game, after he headed the ball he felt a sharp pain in his neck for a short time. He carried on playing but left the pitch 15 min before the game finished as he felt he was getting tired and was having dizzy spells. On the way back home he felt dizzier, sat down and then resumed his walk home. When he arrived at home he felt that his legs were not there and told his father, who came to see him, asked him to stand and found that he could not. When a paramedic team arrived, they found him lying flat on the sofa, not able to move his limbs and complaining of headache. He started complaining of shortness of breath and his O_2 Sat level was 85% in air. O_2 was given and he was strapped onto a trolley and transferred to hospital. On arrival he was given 10 L/min of O_2 via a facemask with a reservoir and the Sat level reached 91%. He is responding to commands but then goes back to sleep. He was electively intubated and ventilated. He is an otherwise fit, young boy who wants to be a sailor. His father has a valvular heart murmur, which was diagnosed at the age of 45 years; he is stable now and does not need any treatment. The boy sometimes gets bruises easily; this was investigated and no abnormality could be found, even with an extended clotting screen. Later he was rushed for an MRI scan, which shows possible left cerebral infarction.

ECHO   Normal heart structure and function
CT brain   No cerebral oedema or bleeding

1. What abnormality is visible on this angiograph?

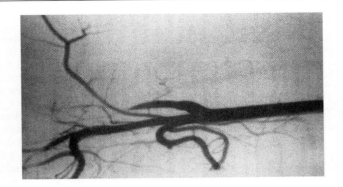

2. What other tests should be carried out?
    a   Cranial MRI
    b   Carotid angiography
    c   DW imaging MRI scan
    d   Thrombophilia screen
    e   ANA
    f   AAs
    g   Sickle-cell screen
    h   Carotid artery Doppler US scan on left side
2. What are the most likely diagnoses?
    a   Dissecting right carotid artery
    b   Right carotid artery aneurysm
    c   Takayasu's disease
    d   Vasculitis
    e   Ehlers–Danlos syndrome
    f   Marfan syndrome
    g   Moyamoya disease
    h   Right carotid artery aneurysm

ANSWERS 81–90

Case 81

1. a   FBC
    c   Blood film
    h   Blood culture
    b   CXR
2. g   ALL
3. d   Hyperhydration
    e   Oral allopurinol
    l   Arrange transfer to specialist unit
    g   No transfusion if there is no mucous membrane bleeding
    a   i.v. antibiotics if febrile

Acute lymphoblastic leukaemia (ALL)

ALL is common between the ages of 2 and 5 years. The cause of leukaemia is not clear but there are certain factors that may increase the risk of developing it, including women being exposed to X-rays during pregnancy, and exposure to nuclear radiation or radiotherapy treatment. Type B lymphoblastic leukaemia is the commonest form to occur in children. The incidence of leukaemia is increased in children with Down syndrome, aplastic anaemia, Turner syndrome, ataxia telangiectasia and Bloom syndrome, and those who have been exposed to certain chemicals. The presentation is varied but usually there is a history of recurrent bruises, painful bones or hips, severe infection, haemorrhage, lymphadenopathy, hepatosplenomegaly, and anaemia. More than 99% of children with leukaemia will have blasts on blood film, with anaemia and neutropenia. A bone marrow analysis will confirm the diagnosis, and information can be gained about the type of leukaemia with cytochemistry and immunological studies. The CSF should be examined, as CNS metastasis is always present. Before starting any treatment, blood should be taken for genetic and immunological study. A blood transfusion should not be given before this. The first step of treatment is to hyperhydrate the patient by giving fluids in the quantity of 2.5 L/m^2 of body surface area. Allopurinol should be given to prevent urate deposition in the kidneys. If the child is febrile and neutropenic, antibiotics should be given. All other advance testing can be carried out in a regional unit with more family support. Treatment should start according to the stage and type of leukaemia. Complications of treatment will arise, and shared care between the local hospital and regional unit will help to overcome these problems.

Case 82

1. a   Sleep EEG
    d   White cell enzyme
    h   Serum AAs
2. f   Non-ketotic hyperglycinaemia

Non-ketotic hyperglycinaemia

This is an inborn error of AA catabolism, causing accumulation of glycine in fluids. Most patients die during the neonatal period if it is very severe, and those who survive are severely retarded and epileptic. It is inherited as an autosomal recessive disorder and antenatal diagnosis can be done by enzymatic assay from fresh chorionic villi biopsy in high-risk groups of patients. The most striking feature is a lack of myelination. The mechanism of neurological dysfunction is poorly understood. Glycine is an inhibitory neurotransmitter with receptors located mainly in the brainstem and spinal cord. This explains only poorly the seizures experienced by these patients, as these seizures arise mainly from the brainstem, and are the main feature of this illness. NMDA receptors are also potentiated by glycine, and excessive activation of these receptors may result in neurotoxicity. The earliest presentation may be 7 hours postdelivery as the neonate exhibits hypotonia and shallow breathing, followed by apnoeic spells. The affected baby will be flaccid and unresponsive, with myoclonic and partial seizures. There is no ketoacidosis, hyperlactataemia or hyperammonaemia. The EEG will show burst suppression, which is an important diagnostic feature. The MRI will show progressive brain atrophy and demyelination. The majority of affected infants will die early and no treatment will be helpful. Those with the infantile type, which is called static encephalopathy, usually will have had a normal birth and an uneventful neonatal period. They are usually developmentally delayed with upper motor neuron signs, poor coordination, expressive speech problems, hyperactivity and aggressive behaviour as well as tonic–clonic seizures. Viral and other illnesses may exacerbate the affected individual's state, making it difficult to control seizure activity. Late onest non-ketotic hyperglycinaemia is very rare and presents with spinocerebellar degeneration and optic atrophy. Levels of plasma and CSF glycine are high, as are those of the glycine CSF/plasma ratio. An enzymatic assay on liver cells or transformed lymphoblasts is the confirmatory test. There is no specific treatment, but supportive treatment in acute deterioration and control of seizures will help the child at school and with mobility.

Case 83

1. g   Blood glucose
2. b   Seizures secondary to hypocalcaemia
3. d   Mother's serum calcium level
   c   Mother's parathyroid hormone level
   j,i Baby's vitamin D and alkaline phosphatase levels

Neonatal hypocalcaemia

This is one of the commonest causes of neonatal seizures among Asian newborn babies. It is usually caused by maternal factors – the mother has a poor calcium intake and the baby suffers from low calcium in utero as well as after birth. Other investigations will be normal. Usually the affected baby will not manifest rickets but will have a low vitamin D level and a high alkaline phosphatase level, which should normalise when the hypocalcaemia is treated. The parathyroid hormone level will be high in these babies and mothers, but this will be normalised by correcting the hypocalcaemia. Dietary assessment for the mother is required in these circumstances, with a multidisciplinary nutritional approach. The mother also needs to take vitamin D as well as a calcium supplement. The prognosis is very good and there are no long-term problems.

Case 84

1. c   Immunoglobulin level
    d   Antibody for pertussis and Hib vaccine
    j   Lymphocyte subset
    b   MRI of right knee
2. a   X-linked agammaglobulinaemia
    b   SCID
    f   SLE

X-linked agammaglobulinaemia (Bruton's disease)

There is a defect in the B-cell line in which pre B-cells fail to differentiate into more mature B-cells. The gene is on the long arm of the X chromosome. Recurrent gynogenic infection in the first year of life will indicate that there is an immunological problem. Pulmonary infection is the most common one, but arthritis, osteomyelitis and gastroenteritis may be the presenting features. Recovery from viral infection is normal but bacterial infections are usually recurrent and it may take 2–3 years to get the correct diagnosis. There will be a normal T-cell pattern but the antibody level in response to vaccines is zero. This usually occurs when the infant is around 4–6 months of age, when the mother's antibodies that crossed the placenta are wearing off. The measurement of IgG will be low. Regular immunoglobulin replacement is needed and the survival rate is improving. Investigation of children with possible immunodeficiency can be very difficult, as infants and children are more vulnerable to viral as well as bacterial infection because of mixing in school. If there is a family history of immunodeficiency, then investigating those children is important in preventing chronicity and early death from severe infection. Children with unusual or opportunistic infection, recurrent minor infection, more than one episode of severe infection, and recurrent infection with allergy or autoimmune disorders are at high risk and should be investigated for possible immune deficiency problems.

Case 85

1. d   Brucellosis
2. e   *Brucella*-specific antibody screen
3. Tetracycline

Undulant fever (brucellosis)

There are three types of organisms that can cause brucellosis, namely are *B. abortus*, *B. melitensis* and *B. suis*. These organisms are primarily diseases of domestic animals such as goats, pigs and cattle, and infection is usually transmitted to humans by ingestion of infected milk and milk products. In infected individuals, there is widespread reticuloendothelial system hyperplasia, especially in the liver and spleen. In chronic infection, the organism will remain intracellular and symptoms develop slowly over a course of months. In the acute phase, symptoms may develop in days with fever, rigors and arthralgia with profuse sweating. The child will look very ill and lose weight rapidly. In chronic forms, the affected child will exhibit fatigue, myalgia, irritability and on/off intermittent fever. Headache and pain everywhere is another feature of chronic brucellosis. It may lead to meningitis, encephalitis, pericarditis and peritonitis, which can be life-threatening. The diagnosis can be confirmed by positive blood culture, but the organism is very difficult to culture. IgM and IgG antibodies can be tested by an agglutination test and this may be positive in asymptomatic patients in highly endemic areas. Increasing titres are diagnostic. In chronic brucellosis, bone marrow, liver, spleen or bone biopsy may be necessary to diagnose this condition. Co-trimoxazole, rifampicin or streptomycin either alone or in combination will be very helpful. In chronic brucellosis, tetracycline is the drug of choice to eradicate chronic infection, but the side-effect profile will not allow its use in children. Rifampicin is the drug of choice as it is the only antibiotic that will eradicate intracellular infection, but resistance to this drug develops very quickly.

Case 86

1. Restrictive and obstructive lung diseases
2. Anterior mediastinal mass
   Tracheal placement to the right
3. c   Spiral chest and abdomen CT
   b   Lateral CXR
4. a   T-cell lymphoma
   c   Teratoma
   b   Thymoma
5. b   Hyperhydration
   e   Allopurinol
   k   Transfer to specialist unit
   m   Bone marrow biopsy
   l   Tissue biopsy from mediastinal mass
   j   Blood for karyotyping and immunological and chemical studies
   o   Save serum
   n   Start dexamethasone after all investigations
   p   Repeat lung function test before travel

Lymphocytic lymphoma

The commonest presentation associated with lymphocytic lymphoma is a mediastinal mass, which can be associated with dyspnoea, superior vena cava obstruction and upper airway obstruction, as in this case. It may also be associated with dysphagia and pleural effusion. Lymph node involvement is usually localised and is mainly located in the neck and axillary region. Liver enlargement with involvement of bone marrow is present in more than 50% of cases and is quite common at the time of presentation. Skin and bone involvement will show mature T-cell lymphocytes. Children with this should have a chest as well as an abdominal CT or MRI. The lung function test is very important, as it will be very helpful in making arrangements for transport and follow-up management. A tissue biopsy from the mediastinal mass is the diagnostic test, and can differentiate this lymphoma from other lymphomas and help in treatment and prognosis. A lumbar puncture should be performed, and a bone scan if bone is involved. LDH should be tested, as it is valuable as a prognostic factor in B-cell disease. A liver, renal, and blood profile should be obtained and blood stored for genetic testing and evaluation for possible bone marrow transplantation before a transfusion is given to these patients (or any oncology patients at first presentation). Surgical resection for a primary mediastinal mass is contraindicated with lymphocytic lymphomas. Intensive chemotherapy with multiagents has increased the survival rate to 80%. Radiotherapy is also helpful, especially when there is CNS involvement.

Case 87

1. c   Dermatomyositis
2. d   CK
    e   LDH
    c   EMG
    b   Muscle biopsy
    a   Thigh muscle MRI
3. a   Oral steroids for 6 months
    f   Physiotherapy
    i   OT (Occupational therapy)

Dermatomyositis

Childhood dermatomyositis is a relatively homogeneous condition that may be caused by a single disease, although not as in adults, in which one-third of cases are associated with malignancy. The illness is usually insidious but can be acute. The individual affected by the insidious form can present with fatigue, fever and anorexia, without any weakness or rash at this stage. In most affected children, involvement of the skin (dermatitis) will develop before involvement of the muscles (myositis). The typical rash is an erythematous discoloration and oedema of the upper eyelids that spreads to involve the entire periorbital and molar area of the face. Erythema and oedema of the extensor surfaces overlying the joints and knuckles, elbows, and knees develop later. The skin looks atrophic and scaly. As symptoms persist, muscle weakness will start to emerge, mainly proximally with pain and stiffness. As the weakness spreads and becomes generalised, joint contractures develop rapidly and produce joint deformities. Subcutaneous calcinosis is not a very good sign and can be very painful. More than two-thirds of affected children will get this, and it can produce more stiffness and pain. Vasculitis in GIT is a predisposing factor of GIT infarction, which has been a leading cause of death in the past. The CK is usually high and an EMG will show increased insertion activity, fibrillation, positive sharp waves at rest, and brief small-amplitude polyphasic potentials with contraction. The muscle biopsy will show perivascular atrophy, which is a diagnostic feature. Corticosteroids will suppress inflammation and relieve symptoms, and can cure dermatomyositis. For treatment of dermatomyositis, a course of corticosteroids should be continued for 2 years. After initial response and 3 months on high-dose corticosteroids, alternating the day with the same dose should continue for 2 years. Physiotherapy is an essential part of treatment and surgical removal of calcinosis can be done if the patient is not responding to corticosteroids, but this cannot always be performed. More than 80% of these patients will have a good prognosis if high-dose corticosteroids are started early. When the disease has become inactive, it is unlikely to become active again. Serum creatinine kinase is one way to monitor response to treatment and activity of the disease.

Case 88

1. h   Toddler's diarrhoea
   f   CMPI
   g   Lactose intolerance
2. e   Nothing

Toddler's diarrhoea

This is characterised by chronic diarrhoea with recognisable undigested food in the stools in a child who is otherwise well, growing, and gaining weight satisfactorily. It usually occurs in toddlers but may occur during the first year of life and progress to childhood. It is a self-limiting illness and no cause can be found. The intestinal postprandial activity is abnormal, and rapid transit of the small intestine may be the cause of this problem. It is one of the commonest reasons for referrals to the paediatrician. Affected children develop normally and there are no signs of FTT, but there is a history of chronic continuous or intermittent diarrhoea. It usually stops between the ages of 2 and 4 years. The pattern usually involves the passing of large, formed or semi-formed faeces early in the day followed by the passing of small amounts of lost stool containing undigested vegetables and mucus. The diagnosis can usually be made on clinical grounds but in cases of doubt and a clinical history that has changed, an intestinal biopsy may be carried out. Reassurance and explanation to the parents of the nature of this condition is very important and no medication is needed. Changing the diet is also not needed.

Case 89

1. a   Dilated lateral ventricles
2. a   Non-communicating hydrocephalus

3.   b, TORCH screen
     c, Chromosomal analysis
     d, Refer to neurosurgeon

Communicating hydrocephalus

This is usually secondary to impaired absorption of CSF, meningitis or subarachnoid haemorrhage. In meningeal malignancy, associated brain tumours or leukaemia, choroid plexus papilloma rarely causes communicating hydrocephalus. In achondroplasia, the hydrocephalus occurs as a result of increased venous pressure due to the narrowing of venous sinuses in the small posterior fossa, leading to obstruction of venous return from the brain. Benign enlargement of the subarachnoid space or external hydrocephalus is also the cause of communicating hydrocephalus. This may appear as a dilating frontal subarachnoid space on CT, with a widening sylvian fissure and other sulci. Most affected children develop normally.

Non-communicating hydrocephalus

This is usually due to an obstruction in CSF circulation between ventricles to the subarachnoid space, which will cause an increase in pressure and ventricular dilation. Aqueduct stenosis is the most common cause, since the aqueduct has the smallest cross-sectional diameter. Congenital atresia or stenosis can occur on its own, but infection, blood clot and compression by tumours may also lead to non-communicating hydrocephalus. Hydrocephalus can present at birth in an infant with an increasing head circumference. It does not respond to drug therapy, and a ventricular peritoneal shunt is the treatment. Mechanical obstruction and infection are problems with use of the shunt. Relieving the pressure in the brain will give the affected child a chance of some normal development but does not result in a normal child. Development of the affected child's verbal skills will be better than that of their non-verbal skills. Other causes include Chiari malformation, Dandy–Walker malformation, Klippel–Feil syndrome, and a mass lesion.

Case 90

1.   Right carotid artery aneurysm
2.   h   Doppler US scans of carotid arteries on right side
     d   Thrombophilia screen
     f   AAs
     c   DW imaging MRI scan
3.   h   Right carotid artery aneurysm
     a   Dissecting right carotid artery
     b   Right carotid artery thrombosis

Arterial aneurysm

These aneurysms rupture – but only very rarely before the age of 10 years. They are usually present before birth, but are not fully developed. An aneurysm may be associated with aortic coarctaction and cystic kidneys. It tends to occur at the bifurcation of major arteries, at the base of the brain or other sites. If it occurs within the brain, it may present as subarchnoid haemorrhage and can be very severe, with loss of consciousness, tachycardia, hypotension and signs of increased intracranial pressure. The first leak is usually small and causes severe headache, neck stiffness and low-grade fever. The oculomotor nerve is the most likely to be affected by pressure, with disturbances in gaze and papillary reaction. A case of internal carotid artery aneurysm may present with a history of hemiplegia with or without bulbar palsy. Catastrophic haemorrhage will cause death. Most patients die from a bleeding arterial aneurysm, which for 50% of these individuals is a first bleed. Another 30% die in the next 10 years. CT is very good for detecting a cerebral bleed in 95% of cases. MRI or MRA is superior to CT, when available. The CSF is usually bloody. The treatment is supportive, but surgical clipping and excision of the aneurysm in the early stages is essential to prevent a further bleed.

Case 91

A 14-year-old boy with a history of lower limb pain for the last 13 months was seen in a paediatric outpatient department. The pain started after a long game of football. Since then he has been complaining of pain in his legs, mainly muscular, and sometimes in his left shoulder and arms. The pain does not wake him up at night and analgesia of any sort is not very helpful. The pain is sharp and worse when he walks; sometimes he loses his balance and falls. He stopped going to school 4 weeks ago as he finds it very difficult to go upstairs for a chemistry session. He admitted that there was bullying at the school last year but not this year. The school headmaster was pleased with his achievement last year. He lives with his mother; his father left home when the boy was 4 years old. The father married in Bangladesh and the boy has never met him. The boy's mother is very anxious and wants him to have a wheelchair so he can go to school, as he will soon be taking GCSE exams.

He is a tall boy and is helped by his mother to walk to the clinic. He is able to take his shoes and trousers off and sit on the bed without a problem. The pain is mainly in his right leg, when touching or bending his right knee. This pain is felt less on the left side and there is evidence of redness or difference in temperature between the calf muscle and thighs. He said that occasionally his left foot and leg get numb and turn blue in colour. All reflexes are intact and the results of a full CNS examination, and a systemic and general examination were normal. Other test results are:

X-rays of lower limbs	No abnormalities
ESR	13 mm/hour
CRP	5
Hb	14.5 g/dl
WCCs	8×10^9/l
PLT	270×10^9/l
LFT, U&E, Ca, phosphate, Mg	All within normal range
TFT, ANA, DNA double strand and rheumatoid factors	Normal
CK	33 mmol/l
EMG, NCS, EEG	Normal

All tests were repeated on three occasions and all test results were normal

1. What is the most likely diagnosis?
    a Post-trauma pain
    b Chronic fatigue syndrome
    c MS
    d Spinal cord compression
    e Becker's disease
    f Dermatomyositis

    g   Reflex sympathetic dystrophy

2.   How should this case be managed?
    a   Simple analgesia
    b   Physiotherapy
    c   Encourage use of a wheelchair
    d   Family therapy
    e   Propranolol
    f   Guanethidine
    g   Referral to pain management team

3.   Which two further tests should be carried out?
    a   Thermography for legs
    b   Doppler study for legs
    c   ANA
    d   DNA double strand
    e   Biopsy of small arteries
    f   Positive emission tomography (PET) scan for legs
    g   Arterial angiography for legs
    h   Venogram for legs

Case 92

A GP who saw a 10-year-old boy referred him as he had had episodes of rectal bleeding, which happened over the weekend, while he was at his friend's house. He went to the toilet and after emptying his bowel, he felt pain and when he looked, there was fresh blood on the toilet seat. By the time he had arrived at the hospital, the bleeding had stopped 3 hours before. He said he got constipated from time to time but this had not happened in the last 6 months. He had never had a bleed before and he does not need to strain while opening his bowel. He looks well, has no rash, fissures or external haemorrhoids. His abdomen is soft and there is no faecal loading or other masses. Investigations were carried out for a possible clotting problem and nothing abnormal was found. He was observed for 24 hours and discharged with a follow-up appointment. He was also referred to an ophthalmologist because of a squint. He was seen by the ophthalmologist, who diagnosed latent squint and also reported that he has retinal pigmented epithelia, which his father also has. The boy has no other illnesses and is generally healthy. An abdominal US, ESR and FBC are normal. He returned to the A&E department with another small bleed and was admitted for further investigations.

1.   What other tests, in order, would help the diagnosis?
    a   Lower GIT endoscopy with biopsies
    b   Meckel scan
    c   Upper GIT endoscopy
    d   Barium swallow and follow-through
    e   Stool culture
    f   Mantoux test
    g   CXR

h   Viral serology
i   Chromosomal study
j   Bone marrow aspirate
k   Sweat test
2.   What is the most likely diagnosis?
a   Peutz–Jeghers syndrome
b   Ulcerative colitis
c   Pseudopolyposis
d   Familial adenomatous polyposis
e   Colonic haemangiomas
f   Meckel's diverticulum
g   Intestinal TB
h   Intestinal lymphoma
i   Intussusception equivalent syndrome
j   Duodenal ulcer

Case 93

A baby girl, now aged 3 weeks, has a correct gestational age of 31 weeks. She tolerates her feed very well via NGT, has a mottled look, tachycardia and tachypnoea. The Sat level is 100% O_2 via a nasal cannula; the CPAP pressure is 5 and flow of 10 L/min is 91%. Her abdomen is distended and soft. She was acidotic (metabolic) with a base deficit of –11. The NGT aspirate was not clear, with slight blood staining. The stool was found on testing to be black, with blood. She was treated with antibiotics and put on i.v. fluid. She was born at 28 weeks' gestation by emergency caesarean section due to prepartum haemorrhage. She was ventilated for 7 days, with maximum support of HFO and conventional ventilation. She developed IVH with right–left ventricular dilatation. She is totally fed on expressed breast milk from her mother, which is tolerated very well. During this episode, the test results are:

Na	128 mmol/l
K	4.1 mmo/l
Ur	8.4 mmol/l
Cr	60 mmol/l
Ca (corrected)	1.99 mmol/l
Phosphate	1.83 mmol/l
Alk. Ph	350 IU/l
ALT	28 IU/l
Alb	32g/l
Hb	9.2 g/dl
WCC	9.3×10^9/l
PLT	350×10^9/l
CRP	30
INR	1.2
PTT	56 s
PT	11 s

1.   What is the immediately required management of this baby girl?

    a Ventilation
    b Abdominal X-ray
    c CXR
    d Repeat head US
    e Change antibiotics
    f Discuss with paediatric surgical team for early transfer
    g Continue feeding
    h Give diuretic
    i Transfer to specialist centre
    j Half correct acidosis with THAM
    k Give i.v. morphine infusion
    l Add metronidazole
    m i.v. fluid with additive (Na, K, Ca)

2.   What two abnormalities are visible on the abdominal X-ray?

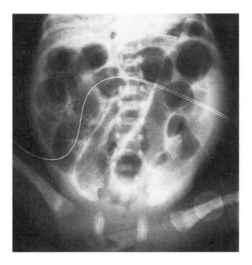

Case 94

A 2-year-old boy presented with a 2-day history of a distended abdomen and puffy eyes. He has vomited several times, his abdomen has become increasingly distended and he has 'white floating stools'. He is passing less urine than normal but hasn't passed any blood. He is not eating and drinking well. He has been very miserable, uncooperative, agitated, and is not himself. A systolic murmur, grade 2/6, is heard more on the left pericardium. He has no history of medication and there is no history of allergies, and he had a normal birth and developmental history. He has poor peripheral perfusion with a HR of 120 b.p.m., a BP of 105/78 mmHg and a RR of 32/min. His abdomen is distended and tense. He is dull to percussion, especially on the flank, which is indicative of fluid in the peritoneal cavity. Other test results are:

Na	127 mmol/l
Alb	11 mmol/l
Cholesterol	7.86
Urine protein	++++
Microscopy	Negative
WBC	5200
CXR	Fluid in transverse fissure on right and patchy right heart border

An ECHO shows a small ASD. A mild vascular rash has appeared on his body in the last 24 hours.

1. What is the most likely diagnosis?
   a   Chickenpox
   b   Nephrotic syndrome
   c   Hepatitis
   d   Heart failure
   e   Peritonitis
   f   UTI
   g   Post-streptococcal glomerular nephritis
2. Which other tests, in order, will help the diagnosis?
   a   24-hour urine collection for proteinuria
   b   Urine C/S
   c   LFT
   d   Viral serology for hepatitis A, B, and C
   e   Abdominal US
   f   ASO titres
   g   Varicella zoster IgM
   h   Lesion swab for virology

Case 95

A 9-month-old boy of mixed race, a twin, was seen at the age of 4 months, with eczema. Treatment in the form of emulsified creams was prescribed. The eczema was present 4 weeks later, with a non-blanching rash at the same time. A diagnosis of infected eczema was made, antibiotics were prescribed and he recovered well. By the age of 7 months, his right eardrum perforated and he was diagnosed as having secretory otitis media. The causative organism is *Staphylococcus aureus*. He also presented at the age of 8 months with diarrhoea, which resolved. He was born at 36 weeks' gestation, after labour was induced due to maternal cholestasis. He was delivered using vantouse, with an Apgar score of 8 at 1 min and no problems at the postnatal check. His twin brother has similar problems, with discharging ears, eczema and perineal abscess. Both boys showed neutropenia and a low platelet count with normal LFT and U&Es. The levels of IgG, A and E are raised. A lymphocyte subset basic panel shows a low T-lymphocyte count; the anti-platelet antibody level was slightly raised and an anti-neutrophil antibody test was negative.

1. What is the most likely diagnosis?
    a   HIV infection
    b   AIDS
    c   SCID
    d   Wiskott–Aldrich syndrome (WAS)
    e   Hypergammaglobulinaemia
    f   Acute lymphoblastic leukaemia
    g   Acute myeloblastic leukaemia
    h   Secondary immune deficiency
    i   Aplastic anaemia
    j   Septicaemia
    k   Histocytosis (Langerhans' disease)
2. Outline an appropriate management plan in order
    a   Regular oral antibiotics
    b   Regular immunoglobulin transfusions
    c   Avoid immunisation with live vaccines
    d   Bone marrow transplant
    e   Physiotherapy
    f   Genetic counselling
    g   Refer to specialist centre for further testing
    h   Withhold all immunisation
    i   Start oral prednisolone
    j   Start antifungal treatment
    k   Regular eczema treatment with emulsified creams and
        hydrocortisone creams

Case 96

A baby was born at 38 weeks' gestation, cephalic, and no
resuscitation was required. His weight was 2.3 kg and height only
41 cm. The OFC was 35 cm. He was fed immediately and his blood
sugar was 2.8 mmol/l at 1 hours of age. He was irritable and it was
noticed that he was more sleepy when another blood sugar test was
carried out; the results were 2.1 mmol/l. Another feed was offered but
the baby was not interested. An NGT was inserted and he was given
40 ml of milk, half of which he vomited straightaway. A septic screen
was carried out, including a lumbar puncture, which was reported as
normal. A high dose of benzylpenicillin and gentamicin was started
and he was kept nil by mouth. A solution of 10% dextrose i.v. fluid
was given at a rate of 9 ml/h when he was aged 4 hours. A quantity of
2 ml/kg of 10% dextrose was given as a bolus, and his blood glucose
was maintained between 2.6–3 mmol/l over the next 12 hours. He
remained irritable, sleepy and lethargic. His serum bilirubin is
150 μmol/l at the age of 24 hours, his Hb is 21 g/dl, platelets 100 ×
10^9/l and CRP < 5. Tests for U&Es, clotting, TFT and a cranial US were
all reported as normal. Other tests included a liver function test and a
bone profile, which were also reported as normal.

1. What is the single most important test that should be carried out?
    a   Blood glucose

    b   PCV
    c   Reticulcytic count
    d   Magnesium
    e   EEG
    f   TORCH screen
    g   Urine culture
    h   CXR
    i   Blood gas
    j   NH$_4$
    k   Lactate
    l   Urine toxicology screen
2. What is the most likely diagnosis?
    a   Sepsis
    b   HIE
    c   Polycythaemia
    d   Hypoglycaemia
    e   Cerebral infarct
    f   Seizures

Case 97

An infant presented to his GP as his parents are very concerned that he is not gaining much weight. The GP said the infant should see a specialist and gave a diagnosis of FTT, with abnormal stools. Three weeks previously, he was admitted with a chest infection, which he recovered from very quickly. During that admission he was found to be neutropenic and a blood test was not repeated as this had contributed to the chest infection. He looks pale, miserable and his weight is only 3.5 kg (birthweight 2.95 kg). His skin is very dry and scaly. His nappy was full, with a very soft, loose and pale stool, which has continued since birth (he is now 2 months old). His chest was clear and no other abnormalities were found on systemic examination. He is taking antibiotics, which were prescribed by his GP for a chest infection. He is anaemic, with a haemoglobin level of 6.7 g/dl, and is neutropenic, with a low platelet count. The results of a CXR and sweat test were reported as normal. The serum immunoglobulin was tested and is within the normal range. HIV antibodies were not detected. The stool has an increased amount of fat, with the presence of positive reducing substance. Results of a blood film and bone marrow test show no evidence of blast cells. The upper GIT endoscopy with biopsy shows no evidence of enteropathies.

1. What is the most likely diagnosis?
2. What other tests should be carried out?
3. What is the prognosis?

Case 98

A 13-year-old girl with a history of rapid weight loss in the last 12 months was referred by her GP. She was an FTND, without neonatal problems. At the age of 3 years, she was admitted with a history of febrile convulsion secondary to tonsillitis, which was treated and did not cause more seizures. At the age of 10 years, while she was on a school trip, the bus collided with another car and she suffered a leg injury, which required tendon repair on her left knee, and she recovered completely. She was doing well at school last term but this term she gets very upset, and says that she does not want to go to school as she feels tired. Her appetite is declining but she is still eating three meals a day, with the family. Following each meal she will go to her room and stay until the next meal, or if there is no meal she will sleep. She said she never eats at school and occasionally she will visit her friend and have a meal with her friend's family. Her mother also said that the girl likes to cook. Her weight is only 27 kg and the results of a systemic and general examination are normal. The results of a FBC, serum electrolytes, liver function, urine, stool, ESR, and CRP are all within the normal range. The CSR and abdominal US results are normal. The blood gas, lactate, NH_4 tests are also normal, as are those for blood glucose, thyroid function, and coeliac screen. The body mass index (BMI) is less than 15.

1. What are the most likely diagnoses?
2. What other tests should be carried out?
3. What is the inheritance pattern?

Case 99

A 13-month-old boy was brought to the Casualty department with a history of drowsiness, irritability and diarrhoea. He has been unwell for the last 2 days, with diarrhoea and temperature. His irritability is worsening, and he is very jittery and clinging to his mother's breast all the time. He was an FTND and there were no neonatal problems. Both parents are from north Africa, are second cousins and have two older boys who are well and thriving. There is no history of miscarriage, or of any family illnesses. The child looks drowsy and dehydrated, and has a HR of 120/min and a RR of 26/min. The CRT is 3 s peripherally and he responds to pain and opens his eyes to his mother's voice. He was taken to the resuscitation room, i.v. access was established and blood was taken and sent to the laboratory for analysis. A quantity of 20 ml/kg of 0.9 normal saline was given over 30 min and he was admitted to the ward. He was treated as having encephalitis, with two antibiotics and aciclovir. The blood results for FBC, U&Es, LFT, CRP, ESR, NH_4, and lactate are normal. The test for arterial blood gas (ABG) shows mild metabolic acidosis, which may be related to dehydration. A lumbar puncture shows no abnormalities and the PCR for herpes simplex virus was negative. The antibiotics and aciclovir were stopped and he was discharged home on the 5th day of admission, although his mother said he is still not 100% back to normal. Two days after discharge, his mother brought him to Casualty, saying that he cannot speak and is moving his arms a lot. He had dystonic movement, affecting the arms, body and tongue. He is not able to sit any more and finds it very difficult to feed. He was admitted as seizures were possible, diagnosis of dystonia was made and rectal diazepam was given, which stopped all movement but made him more sleepy. A cranial CT and urgent EEG were carried out and reported as normal. The two antibiotics were started again as well as aciclovir, which were to finish in 1 week and 2 weeks, respectively. Blood was sent for *Mycoplasma* titres, herpes viruses IgG, and repeated metabolic screen including AAs, and urine for AAs and organic acids. He continues to have abnormal movements when he wakes up and is not able to sit or stand, which he used to do. The urine organic acid test shows an abnormally high level of glutaric, 3-hydroxyglutaric, 3-hydroxybutyric and acetoacetic acids. His repeated MRI scan shows an increased signal in the basal ganglia and attenuation in the white matter. He was started on Sinemet (co-careldopa) on a trial dose, which he tolerated well, and the movements in his arms and legs were reduced. The plan is to increase the dose slowly over the next 3 months.

1. What other investigations may help the diagnosis?
2. What is the most likely diagnosis?
   a Encephalitis
   b Partially treated meningitis
   c Neuroblastoma
   d Meningoencephalitis
   e Reye syndrome
   f Glutaric aciduria type 1
   g Urea cycle defect
   h Drug toxicology
   g Methylmalonic aciduria
   h Brain tumour
3. What should the parents be told?

Case 100

A male infant was seen in A&E with a history of being unwell with a high temperature. He is 4 months old, is completely uninterested in food, and is very irritable and crying. This has been going on for the last 48 hours. There is no rash on his body and he was last fed 8 hours ago. His neck is hyperextended, even when the temperature has come down. He is fully vaccinated, including for *Haemophilus influenzae* and *Neisseria meningitidis* class C. He was born by full-term vaginal delivery and there were no neonatal problems. There are no illnesses in the family; his mother is only 17 years old and his father of a similar age. He was given ibuprofen, i.v. access was established and antibiotics were given. He was given resuscitation fluid and put on dextrose/saline maintenance fluid. His LP shows evidence of bacterial meningitis and no organism was isolated. On day 5, he continued to spike a temperature but was less irritable, with a bulging fontanelle. He is well perfused and is feeding well. His inflammatory marker is coming down but his WCC is still high. On day 6 he is still not right and another antibiotic is added. On day 7 he is still spiking a temperature, up to 38°C, and has a bulging fontanelle. A cranial US scan was reported as normal and a repeated LP shows only a few white cells, high protein and normal glucose levels.

1. What is the most useful other test?
   a   CSF PCR for *Pneumococcus*, H. *influenzae* and *N. meningitides*
   b   CSF PCR for virology
   c   CSF PCR for mycobacteria
   d   Cranial CT with contrast
   e   CXR
   f   HIV testing
   g   Mantoux test
   h   *Mycoplasma* titres
2. What is the most likely diagnosis?
   a   Tuberculous meningitis
   b   Subdural effusion
   c   Space-occupying lesion
   d   Partially treated meningitis
   e   Viral encephalitis
   f   Hydrocephalus

ANSWERS 91–100

Case 91

1.   g   Reflex sympathetic dystrophy (RSD)
2.   a   Simple analgesia
     b   Physiotherapy
     d   Family therapy
     g   referral pain management team
3.   a   Thermography for legs
     g   Arterial angiography for legs

Reflex sympathetic dystrophy

This is characterised by severe pain in the limbs with vasomotor and pseudomotor dysfunction, leading to atrophic changes in skin, muscle and bone, following trauma. Trauma can be incidental or surgical. It is more common in girls in their early teens. The injury can be slight and symptoms are usually not specific for the first 3–4 months. The pain usually starts at the site of injury and spreads proximally or distally without any specific landmark or dermatome. There is usually a swelling of the affected side, with vasomotor changes in the majority of cases. Pain is usually burning or aching and exacerbated by movement or dependence; this may cause an arm or leg to be held in a certain position, which may lead to muscle atrophy. There is no specific timing for this pain, and specific tests can be carried out. The thermograph as well as Doppler to analyse circulation may show a decrease in perfusion as a blue area. The PET scan will help to detect areas of reduced perfusion. Angiography is less desirable as the results are not as good as for the tests mentioned earlier. In general children do better than adults – 50% of affected children recover within the first year and the rest will recover later, but there are no long-term problems. Patients should be treated with analgesia, guanethidine (propranolol – nerve block) and sympathectomy. Psychiatric and physiotherapy support is very important in these cases.

Case 92

1. a   Lower GIT endoscopy with biopsies
   i   Chromosomal study
   d   Barium swallow and follow-through
2. d   Familial adenomatous polyposis

Familial adenomatous polyposis

This condition is inherited as an autosomal dominant trait and usually starts to cause problems after puberty, but many cases present early, before puberty. It is characterised by diarrhoea, blood and mucousy stools. The child who presents with blood or mucus in the stool without any evidence of inflammatory bowel disease, constipation or infective diarrhoea should be suspected of having polyps. Children with a family history of polyposis should be offered genetic testing. The gene is located on chromosome 5q21. Regular colonoscopies should be performed after the affected child reaches the age of 10 years. The treatment is total colectomy in early adulthood to avoid large-bowel malignancy.

Case 93

1. a   Ventilate
   k   Give i.v. morphine infusion
   l   Add metronidazole
   m   i.v. fluid with additive (Na, K, Ca)
   f   Discuss with paediatric surgical team for early transfer
   j   Half correct acidosis with THAM
2. Intramural gas
   Dilated loops

Necrotising enterocolitis

The incidence in premature babies is 3 in 1000 live births as well as some term babies. The median age of onset is GA < 26 weeks: 23 days, GA > 31 wks: 11 days. There is a diffuse and patchy area of mucosal ulceration, oedema and haemorrhage, leading to necrosis within the small or large intestine. It may or may not be associated with perforation. The commonest sites affected are the jejunum, ileum and colon. Any part of the GIT may be affected. It is a transmural disease with distended loops of intestine with spotty intramural haemorrhages, and areas of necrosis may be seen macroscopically. It has been suggested that cytokines have an important role in mediating intestinal inflammation and damage but the exact cause is not yet known. Gut hypoxia is another factor that may be the leading cause of necrotising enterocolitis (NEC). Infection, enteral feeding and some drugs are also risk factors. Formula milk and its early introduction increases the risk of developing NEC 6–10 times more than breast milk; this may be due to mucosal damage by hyperosmolar feeds. Abdominal distension, bloody mucousy stools, and bile-stained aspirates or vomit are the main clinical presentation of this condition. It can be insidious (causing lethargy, temperature instability, apnoea and hypoperfusion).

The symptoms are variable, from feed intolerance to intra-abdominal catastrophe with sepsis, shock, peritonitis and death. Doctors and nurses who are looking after premature babies should be alerted to suspect. NEC in such babies who deteriorate suddenly with no evidence of infection or intraventricular haemorrhage and who are not on a ventilator. There are many signs, including a palpable distended loop, a distended abdomen; change of colour of the abdominal wall from blue to red, changes in blood test results such as leukopenia, anaemia, thrombocytopenia and acidosis, DIC, low sodium level and high urea and creatinine levels. The abdominal X-ray is very helpful but interpretation should be done carefully. Pneumatosis intestinalis is pathognomonic, but thickened intestinal walls with fluid level and dilated loops, a gasless abdomen, and gas in the portal venous system with subdiaphragmatic air are other radiological features associated with NEC. The treatment is supportive, but early surgical intervention to remove the damaged portion of the gut is vital for the survival of the baby. All enteral feeding should be stopped, a free drainage NGT inserted, antibiotics initiated, and acidosis corrected. Ventilation is essential, as well as strong analgesia. Regular head scans can be associated with IVH. The overall mortality rate is 22% without surgery, and post-surgery it goes up to 40%. There is a 10% risk of relapse in the first month. Other problems such as stricture formation occur in more than one-quarter of cases.

Case 94

1. b   Nephrotic syndrome
2. a   24-hour urine collect for proteinuria
   c   LFT
   e   Abdominal US
   h   Lesion swab for virology
   g   Varicella zoster IgM

Nephrotic syndrome

Nephrotic syndrome is characterised by proteinuria > 3 g/24 hours, hypoalbuminaemia < 30g/l, and oedema. Hypercholesterolaemia is almost always present. It can affect those at any age but the peak age for onset is between 1 and 5 years and it is more prevalent in males. Hypoalbuminaemia secondary to heavy proteinuria will lead to an increase in catabolism, limiting the amount of protein in the urine and concealing the extent of protein loss through the glomerula. Structural damage to the glomerular basement membrane causes an increase in the size and number of pores, which can lead to proteinuria. The oedema can be caused by the difference between the onocotic pressure and pressure in afferent glomerular arterioles. Activation of the renin–angiotensin–aldosterone system further exacerbates the oedema. The commonest pathological change associated with nephrotic syndrome is a minimal change, which accounts for 90% of cases in children. Other causes may include systemic vasculitis, (e.g. HSP, SLE) infections, (e.g. malaria) allergens, (e.g. a bee sting) diabetic glomerulosclerosis, amyloidosis, and agents (penicillamine, gold and mercury). The early signs of nephrotic syndrome are periorbital oedema, and scrotal, leg and ankle oedema. Ascites will follow later, accompanied by breathlessness due to pleural effusions and abdominal distension. Medication should include (initial episode) prednisolone 60 mg/m²/day until there is no protein in the urine for 3 days, then change to 40 mg/m²/day on alternate days for 4 weeks. Treatment for 3 months or more will, these days, reduce the chances of relapse in the steroid respondent patients. For the first two relapses, the regimen mentioned earlier should be followed but with frequent maintenance prednisolone 0.1–0.5 mg/kg/alternating days for 3–6 months, then reduced by 5 mg every week. For children who have relapsed while on prednisolone, other drugs should be considered, such as levamisole 2.5 mg/kg/alternating days for 4–12 months or cyclophosphamide 3 mg/kg/d for 8 weeks. Children who have relapsed on prednisolone > 0.5 mg/kg/alternating days could be given cyclosporin A 5 mg/kg/day for 1 year. Prophylaxis with penicillin should be given to all children with relapsed nephrotic syndrome. Some relapsed children may present with hypovolaemia in the form of ascites, abdominal pain, a raised haemoglobin level and PCV, tachypnoea, low blood pressure, and a very tired appearance. Giving i.v. 4.5% albumin 10 ml/kg will help, but if severe oedema is is present, the child should be given 20% albumin 5 ml/kg with frusemide 0.5 mg/kg halfway through the infusion, with careful monitoring of output, BP and electrolytes. If there is no improvement, then the child should be referred to a specialist.

Case 95

1. d   WAS (Wiskott–Aldrich syndrome)
2. a   Regular oral antibiotics

c   Avoid immunisation with live vaccines
g   Refer to specialist centre for further testing
f   Genetic counselling
k   Regular eczema treatment with emulsified creams and
     hydrocortisone

Wiskott–Aldrich syndrome

WAS belongs to a group of combined immunodeficiency syndromes
and involves of a variety of defective mechanisms in lymphocyte
function that tend to have similar clinical features. These clinical
features show opportunistic infections arising as a result of combined
deficiencies in cell-mediated immunity and antibody production. It is
mainly a cell-mediated defect causing a falling level of
immunoglobulin. It is an X-linked recessive disorder characterised by
thrombocytopenia purpura, eczema, and draining ears. The gene is
found on the proximal arm of the X chromosome at Xp11.22. There
are a few genetic mutations associated with WAS, including single
base changes, single codon deletions or insertions, and intronic
mutations. There are other pathological problems associated with
WAS, including platelet abnormality, a defect in dendritic cells,
defects in cell motility, and an abnormal rate of synthesis and
catabolism of Ig and Alb. There is impairment of the humoral
immune response to polysaccharide antigens and poor or absent
antibody responses after immunisation with polysaccharide vaccines.
The presentation can start in the infant as early as 3 months of age,
with prolonged bleeding from a circumcision site, or bloody
diarrhoea. Atopic dermatitis can be the first presentation, with
recurrent infections such as otitis media, pneumonia, meningitis, and
sepsis. *Pneumocystis carinii* and herpesviruses are other
opportunistic infections that may occur.

On clinical examination, eczema is always present, but petechial or
purpuric rashes are not always presenting features. Splenomegaly
and hepatomegaly with cervical lymphadenopathy are other features
associated with WAS. Genetic counselling and prenatal diagnosis is
available. Regular prophylactic antibiotics and vigorous treatment of
infections are necessary. There has been some success with bone
marrow transplants and that is the long-term aim. In some patients,
malignancy can be associated with this syndrome. The mortality rate
from severe sepsis is high.

Case 96

1.   b   PCV
2.   c   Polycythaemia

Polycythaemia

This is characterised by a raised hematocrit level and increased
blood viscosity. There are several causes of polycythaemia,

including placental insufficiency, feto-maternal transfusion, maternal smoking, twin–twin transfusion, maternal diabetes, delayed cord clamping, neonatal thyrotoxicosis, unattended delivery, congenital adrenal hyperplasia, and chromosome abnormalities. Polycythaemia may lead to hypoglycaemia and hyperbilirubinaemia. The affected baby may be asymptomatic, but the risks of hyperviscosity such as respiratory distress, renal artery occlusion, heart failure, cerebrovascular occlusion, platelet consumption, and NEC may rise if this is not treated carefully. A central venous PCV of 65 will indicate polycythaemia, but if the peripheral venous PCV is in the range of 65–70 and the capillary PCV > 70 at 2 hours of age, watch for symptoms and repeat tests before considering treatment. Symptomatic babies with PCV > 70 require exchange transfusion; this should be considered in symptomatic babies with PCV ranging from 65 to 69. Babies with venous PCV > 65 are at risk of hyperviscosity.

Asymptomatic babies need observation only, but babies with symptoms such as jitteriness, irritability or floppiness, or any other neurological signs, should be considered for partial exchange transfusion.

Case 97

1. Schwachman–Diamond syndrome
2. Exocrine pancreatic function test
   Platelet count
   U&E
   Chromosomal study
3. One-quarter of these patients may develop myelodysplastic syndrome

Schwachman–Diamond syndrome

This is not a rare disease and affected individuals usually present with FTT and recurrent chest infections. It is an autosomal recessively inherited disorder. The immunoglobulin is normal but there is cyclic neutropenia, which leads to bacterial infection, mainly in the lungs. A low platelet count is also present in more than two-thirds of patients, which may cause recurrent bruises but rarely leads to catastrophic bleeding. In more than half of affected patients, this can be very severe and is due to bone marrow suppression. The skin is also abnormal, with very dry, scaly and flaky skin, which resolves as the malabsorption is corrected. The exocrine pancreatic function test is abnormal, and the pancreatic insufficiency experienced in this syndrome is similar to that in cystic fibrosis. Replacement therapy is required. The sweat test is negative. The prognosis is not bad if infection can be detected early and treated. Regular check-ups are required and one-quarter of affected patients will develop myelodysplasia.

Case 98

1. Anorexia nervosa
2. Serum U&E
3. Multifactorial

Anorexia nervosa

This is an eating disorder with underlying psychological disturbance and is characterised by a distorted body image, fear of obesity and significant weight loss. It is more common in females and about 1% of females aged 15–30 years will be anorexic. Other features of anorexia nervosa apart from distorted body image are yellowish skin, hypercortisolism, hyperglycaemia, and hypokalaemia. It can lead to many other problems. Some patients need to be admitted and a feeding programme established. Unfortunately mortality still occurs, even when they are sectioned; the suicide rate is very high among these patients.

Case 99

1. Check urine of other siblings for organic acids
2. f   Glutaric aciduria type 1
3. Genetic counselling
   Prenatal diagnosis can be offered
   The child will have motor and cognitive problems in future and his condition may get worse with any infectious disease he may get

Glutaric aciduria

This is a rare metabolic disease with abnormalities in lysine, hydroxylysine and tryptophan metabolism. It is an autosomal recessive disorder and there are two types. Type 1 is usually manifested in the first year of life in infants. The child may present as suffering from an infective illness such as gastroenteritis or a UTI, from which he or she will recover, then start having dystonic movement, hypotonia and dysmetria. The acute encephalitic illness is associated with infection and the infant usually presents with irritability, somnolence and excessive sweating. Seizures may accompany this illness or appear later. Following this the child may develop dystonic movement, and choreoathetosis may also develop. The child's development is starting to regress at this stage. At presentation, blood gas analysis may show metabolic acidosis but there will be an abnormal amount of glutaric, 3-hydroxyglutaric, 3-hydroxybutric and acetoacetic acids in the urine. A definitive diagnosis can be made after a fibroblast culture is taken, looking for specific enzyme deficiency.

A cranial MRI scan will show attenuation of the cerebral white matter and cerebral atrophy. The long-term prognosis is not very good and controlling the movement by dopaminergic drugs and physiotherapy is important. Protein should be excluded from the diet and this will help to reduce the risk of deterioration. Genetic counselling should be offered to the parents, and screening of siblings can be carried out as some symptoms may present late.

Case 100

1. a   PCR for *Neisseria*, *Pneumococcus* and *Haemophilus influenzae* from CSF
2. b   Subdural effusion secondary to meningitis

Postmeningitis subdural effusion

Subdural effusion following meningitis has been increasingly recognised, especially following infection with *H. influenzae* meningitis, and can laterally and mainly occupy the frontoparietal region. After treatment for meningitis, the child can remain febrile and the development of focal neurology may indicate subdural effusion. The cranial CT scan is very good at picking up subdural collection. The fluid usually contains no blood but a lot of protein. If the fontanelle still remains open, it usually bulges and is tense. The ventricle may be dilated and hydrocephalus may arise. If the child's condition deteriorates as a result of increased intracranial pressure, subdural tapping can be carried out through the anterior fontanelle if it is still open or a shunt can be inserted in the subdural space for older children. Most instances of subdural collection following meningitis resolve spontaneously. Other organisms such as *Pneumococcus* and *Neisseria meningitidis* can also cause subdural effusion. Complications may arise, such as hydrocephalus, venous sinus thrombosis, venous infarct and brain abscess.